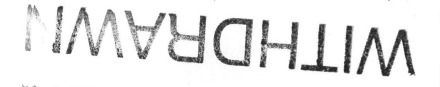

❧

The
STRATEGIC
Health Care
MANAGER

George H. Stevens

The STRATEGIC *Health Care* MANAGER

Mastering Essential Leadership Skills

 Jossey-Bass Publishers

San Francisco

THE STRATEGIC HEALTH CARE MANAGER
Mastering Essential Leadership Skills
   by George H. Stevens

Copyright © 1991 by: Jossey-Bass Inc., Publishers
                    350 Sansome Street
                    San Francisco, California 94104

For sales outside the United States, please contact your local Simon & Schuster
International Office.

Jossey-Bass Web address: http://www.josseybass.com

Library of Congress Cataloging-in-Publication Data

Stevens, George H., date.
   The strategic health care manager : mastering essential leadership
skills / George H. Stevens. — 1st ed.
      p.   cm. — (The Jossey-Bass health series)
   Includes bibliographical references and index.
   ISBN: 978-0-470-63118-8
      1. Health facilities — Administration.   2. Leadership.   I. Title.
II. Series.
      [DNLM: 1. Delivery of Health Care — organization &
administration.   2. Health Facilities — organization & administration.
3. Health Facility Administrators.   4. Leadership.   5. Practice
Management, Medical.   WX 155 S844s]
   RA971.S76   1991
   362.1'068'4 — dc20
   DNLM/DLC
   for Library of Congress   90-15634

JACKET DESIGN BY WILLI BAUM

FIRST EDITION

Code 9125

The Jossey-Bass Health Series

Contents

ix

Preface

With the exception of senior executives and corporate staff, most health care managers have risen through the ranks. These managers, technical experts in one or more of the myriad technical and scientific professions that comprise health care, are the backbone of the provider organization. No plan developed by senior managers, no matter how creative and intelligent, would succeed without the leadership of department heads and other line managers in the provider organization. The middle level of management in today's provider is often the only level at which clinical care and management are unified in a single leadership role. And yet, professionals in these crucial positions are faced with many challenges for which they have not been prepared. These challenges provide both opportunity for unparalleled achievement and the threat of organizational failure. The opportunities and challenges of health care management are the result of two factors:

- Unique forces are dramatically changing the way health care is both managed and delivered.
- The majority of health care managers in America have been expected to master the skills of management on their own.

The first of these factors has been given priority by leaders in the industry, who have adapted their approaches to marketing, capital development, and planning in response to competitive and technological forces unique to the health care industry. But preparing midlevel line managers has not received the attention it requires. This book is for those managers. It is for managers in the nursing, respiratory care, physical therapy, pharmacy, nutrition, social services, facilities, and many other services essential to provider operation. Without these services and the dedication of their managers, no provider could survive.

Little consideration is given to the fact that most health care managers have been trained as technical experts in their scientific and technical disciplines—*not* in the use of influence or in business management. These managers are thrust into positions of administrative leadership because they have demonstrated *clinical* and *technical* leadership.

Experienced clinicians placed in this role quickly realize that life as a manager is replete with at least as many challenges as when they were caring for patients. But these new challenges are very different from providing patient care. This book is for these professionals who embrace management as a second career. It is for managers and future managers who strive to master a suddenly broadened scope of responsibility and completely different set of performance expectations from those learned in professional training.

The Strategic Health Care Manager provides strategies that enable managers to lead by proactively planning for technical, market, and regulatory change and to build a team of professionals fully capable of implementing these plans. These changes affect a provider as significantly as scientific and clinical developments employed in the organization. The book presents proven, systematic approaches to the process of management. It presents a practical but challenging model of leadership in the industry and presents the most important responsibilities of the manager who is also a leader.

This book is *not* a compendium of all the skills a manager will need to succeed in health care, if such a thing were possible.

Nor is it a book about basic principles of management. (There are more than enough of those already.) *The Strategic Health Care Manager* is a guide for developing a proactive management strategy for the most crucial of the many issues facing the modern health care manager. Its mission is to help managers understand the role they can play in leading their organization to success. This mission is important because the manager's job is to lead people, not to administer operations. To be sure, the manager must make certain that operations run smoothly, but that is not the manager's mission. That part of the manager's role is the price to be paid for the excitement, challenge, and reward of being an agent of innovation for his or her organization.

A primary assumption of this book is that a manager is in the greatest of all learning environments—the provider organization. *The Strategic Health Care Manager* distills theory and extensive observations of provider organizations into immediately useful strategy. To this end, readers will find practical and proven approaches for managers who want to achieve sustained excellence in their departments.

The manager's responsibilities were once defined as planning, organizing, staffing, implementing, and evaluating the work of others to accomplish an assigned departmental function. Indeed, this model is still taught in many management courses for health professionals. A revolution in health care over the past ten years has made this view of health care management obsolete. This revolution has altered and continues to alter the technology used to provide care, the ways in which we pay for care, and the role of the middle manager in the success of the provider organization.

The difference between success and failure in health care is increasingly determined by the ability of very diverse professionals to function as a team. While today's health care manager is still responsible for balancing a budget and staffing the night shift, these skills represent only one level of challenge. A greater challenge is the ability to communicate a vision of success and to influence both staff and peers to help make that success a reality. Because of this challenge, many of the skills discussed in the book are addressed with the support of resources that the reader can use immediately.

Management in health care will never again be a profession of administration. It is, and will continue to be, one of savvy marketing by middle managers, design of convenient and caring services for customers who include more than the patient and the physician, and, above all, leadership by example and respect. This book presents tools for managerial success for this new profession.

Overview of the Contents

The book is divided into nine chapters. The first chapter presents an overview of the most significant changes in the health care industry in the past decade and describes how these changes have affected the provider organization and the individual manager. The second chapter presents the most important responsibility of leadership in the health care industry in the face of these industry changes. Each of the chapters from Three through Nine focuses on one critical skill set that must be mastered by the manager who would succeed in today's provider organization. These skills are a far cry from the traditional ones of planning, staffing, controlling, and so on. They are also not found in many allied health or other technical curricula. The highly professional and autonomous nature of most health care professions demands a unique set of management tools.

Chapter One describes the choice faced by today's provider organization. That choice often seems to be one of either providing quality health care or maintaining fiscal viability for a department or an institution. This chapter describes industrial, political, and planning forces that will determine the fate of a manager—forces of little daily consequence to a clinical practitioner. The manager must become acutely aware of these forces, how they affect his departments, and how he can use them to his advantage.

Chapter Two describes the role of the manager in the environment created by the forces described in the first chapter. There are many roles that the manager can assume in today's provider organization. Some of these are comfortable and require the manager to guide daily, weekly, and monthly operations. These roles, however, will lead to stagnation and obsolescence. The chapter defines a desirable leadership role and explains why and how the manager must assume such an aggressive, visionary, and progressive role in an industry steeped in tradition and authority.

Chapter Three focuses on the manager's ability to communicate. Communication, through salesmanship, listening, negotiating, and several other approaches, is essential to successful influence by a manager whose scope of responsibility often exceeds his formal scope of authority.

Chapter Four focuses on the crucial role of planning and a strategic approach to it. It describes characteristics of successful planning and provides a step-by-step model for effective planning at the departmental level. This model directly ties together in a cause-effect process several critical determinants of planning success.

Chapter Five presents a rationale for adopting a model for effective project management in health care management. The rationale is based on empirical evidence from successful health care provider organizations. The chapter further differentiates project management from more traditional functional management and defines the most important components of projects for the manager.

Most, if not all, of the professions allied for the delivery of health care claim a reverence for the "team approach." Yet the reality of modern health care is that its teams are often fragmented and less than effective. Chapter Six describes customer service criteria for evaluating a team, tools for assessing the effectiveness of a team, and strategies for effective team leadership.

Chapters Seven and Eight explore the crucial nature and specific responsibilities of the manager's role in departmental performance effectiveness. Chapter Seven focuses on defining specific activities that the manager must lead to ensure that a department's staff is prepared for both the technical requirements of today's workplace and emerging responsibilities of the industry. The chapter provides a model to help managers ensure peak staff performance by using training as a strategic tool rather than as a benefit for employees.

Because of the essential and changing role played by day-to-day staff performance in the overall effectiveness of a department, Chapter Eight introduces the health care manager to essential principles of performance systems management. The focus of this chapter is on the strategies a manager may use quickly and effectively to improve the performance of staff in most job responsibilities with or without traditional training.

Chapter Nine presents guidance for beginning or continuing the process of becoming a health care strategic manager. It also introduces a case illustration of strategic health care management, presented in Resource D. The example demonstrates how a health care manager can integrate the advice and techniques presented in the book on the job.

Acknowledgments

I am deeply grateful to many people who inspired, motivated, and cajoled me as this book was in development.

Donald N. Lombardi of CHR/Intervista conceived the idea for the book and encouraged me to begin. His hand is at work in other ways, as well. As a mentor, he has shaped my approach to management and human performance for nearly a decade.

I am also indebted to Joseph G. Sorbello, assistant professor of programs in respiratory care and cardiorespiratory sciences at the State University of New York Health Science Center in Syracuse. He provided advice and counsel about the overall manuscript and wrote Chapter Three, "Communicating Effectively."

My gratitude also goes to Jossey-Bass editors Alis Valencia and especially Rebecca McGovern for their patience, gentle encouragement, and constructive criticism as the book evolved.

Reisterstown, Maryland   George H. Stevens
January 1991

The Author

George H. Stevens is a partner in Integrated Performance Designs, which provides services to health care organizations in performance systems design, computer-based systems for performance improvement, management and technical skill training systems design, and competency-based employee development. Stevens's clients include acute and long-term care providers, payors, and health care educational institutions. Stevens received his B.S. degree (1981) from the State University of New York at Upstate Medical Center in respiratory care and his M.S. degree (1983) from Syracuse University in instructional systems design, development, and evaluation.

Stevens has been responsible for the design and development of educational products and systems used for senior management education and by consultants to business and industry and financial management executives. He is a frequent contributor to professional journals and texts, addressing issues of instructional systems design, human peformance systems design, and appropriate application of emerging technologies for performance improvement.

Stevens was formerly associate director of education for the American College of Healthcare Executives, where he was responsible for the design of continuing education curricula for health care executives across the United States and abroad.

*This book is dedicated with gratitude
to the people who help me grow —
people who may not always understand my work,
but who nonetheless believe in me:
Marilyn Margaret, Joshua Richard,
Emily Jane, Laura Elizabeth, Bill,
and always, Richard.*

1

What Every Health Care Manager Faces: *Quality Care Versus Financial Despair*

For some time now, a revolution has been brewing in the technology, utilization, financing, and management strategy of American health care that has dramatically and permanently altered its practice. Rather than slowing after an initial period of growth to allow the industry to adjust to changes, these trends continue to accelerate, creating an environment where change is the only constant in today's health care delivery system. These trends are myriad, affecting such diverse elements as specific treatment modalities used in patient care, the acquisition of capital, strategic planning, and basic organizational structure. The one thread common to all of these changes, however, is that which impacts the role of the keystone of successful health care planning and delivery: the midlevel health care manager. To meet the challenges posed by these trends, managers must make strides on two equally important fronts: acquiring technical skills in the science of business management and developing the attitudes and interpersonal skills needed to be dynamic leaders in a changing business. In this chapter I will attempt to briefly describe the major trends of this industrywide revolution. I will also describe how these trends impact the manager and the effective operation of the provider organization. Finally, I will present an overview of the management skills that will empower

1

health care managers to successfully manage this "revolution," as leaders of positive change in their organizations.

Midlevel health care managers are being called on to assume greater levels of responsibility and more prominent roles in the strategic planning of services and programs for both patients and their families. This calling is due in large part to the unique perspective of the midlevel manager. *Midlevel manager* is necessarily a broadly focused term. Here it refers to all allied health and other managers who have moved into the ranks of management after proving themselves expert in some facet of technical skill application. That skill may be nursing, physical therapy, or any of a host of applied sciences. It is this manager alone who has an intimate understanding of both patient care issues and the realities of managing with extremely limited resources. CEOs and strategic planners, realizing the value of such a perspective, are calling on managers to become more active partners in the management of organizational performance. This will require that managers have a level of creativity and skill never before needed for their jobs. Some of the skills I will present in this book are radically different than those presented in traditional textbooks for health care management. In order to understand this apparent incongruity, a brief explanation of these trends and what they mean for the manager and for the industry is necessary.

Payment Capitation

In the early 1980s there began a trend that changed the way in which the federal government, and later all health care payors, reimbursed providers for patient care services. The federal government, concerned that the cost of providing health care to America's aging population would soon bankrupt the Medicare program, implemented a new method of paying health care providers for care rendered to Medicare patients. Under this elaborate new system, a limit was placed on the amount of money paid to a hospital for treating any specific diagnosis. This limit, or capitation, was determined by the severity of the disease, the age of the patient, the average length of stay (LOS), and other factors.

If a hospital was able to successfully discharge a patient before actually incurring all costs allowed in a payment, then it could "keep the difference and make a profit" on that patient. If a hospital was unable to treat and release a patient before spend-ing the amount of money the government was willing to pay for diagnosed ailments, the hospital was expected to make up the difference from other, more profitable, patient visits. The intent of this reimbursement system was twofold. First, the government hoped to provide an incentive to hospitals to reduce the cost of providing patient care. Second, the reimbursement system (pro-spective payment) was theoretically designed to improve the quality of care provided to America's ill. This would happen through the elimination of unnecessary procedures and inor-dinately long hospitalizations recommended by cautious medi-cal professionals seeking to avoid litigation in malpractice suits.

One development does not a trend make. But the govern-ment's experiment at cost control was very successful, by some measures—so successful, in fact, that most private health insur-ance companies now use some variation of the prospective payment system when determining how much they will pay hospitals and individual professionals for patient care. There are different approaches to prospective payment now, but cap-itation of payment is a feature common to all.

The impact of this change was and continues to be very profound. Prior to capitated payment, health care management strategy was to expand on an annual basis in order to provide services to the entire community, regardless of the profitability of services planned. Under prospective payment, however, health care managers must pay for community health programs from a significantly smaller revenue base. In order to do this, managers must become more selective, prioritizing those ser-vices that are of highest need in the community and those that promise to provide the greatest revenue for future operations. Faced with this threat of reduced ability to expand, managers must develop ways to simultaneously maximize revenue and reduce operating costs in order to make up the deficit created by a curtailment of "cost-plus" payment for services provided. Because of this, providers must evaluate carefully which services they can afford to provide. To do this effectively, developing skills in the technical disciplines of business management is a priority for managers.

Health care managers in practice during the years from 1980–1988 will probably recall the period in terms of the changing emphasis placed on each of these disciplines, as their impact began to be felt on the everyday operations of the provider organization. First, it seems, there was the era of "guest relations," in which entire employee populations were herded into seminar rooms for three days and given a new awareness of the importance of customer satisfaction. This was followed by a brief period of apparent confusion in the industry regarding the roles of public relations, advertising, and marketing, in which each of these three unique disciplines was shouldered with the burden of the other two and ostracized when unable to solve all of the hospitals' census and revenue woes. When this confusion subsided, there was left in place an expanded role for each of these marketing-related disciplines and a new-found appreciation for the power of market-based business strategy development. In the midst of the marketing era, the health care industry became aware of the need for individual fiscal responsibility and focused its collective sights on the containment of cost and optimization of credit ratings as a way to further enhance ability to pay for the patient care needs of the community. This led to a close scrutiny of all capital and payroll expenses, new techniques of cost accounting and day-to-day financial controls. Strategic capital planning became yet another priority for health care organizations that sought to improve their financial position through debt-funded business ventures. These ventures were designed to reduce the provider's dependence on inpatient care as a sole source of revenue. They were often structured as joint ventures in which the provider would enter into a partnership with physicians who would provide medical management and patient referrals in return for equity. Managers were now expected to be conversant in issues of the bond market and financial planning and to be able to identify opportunities for developing new businesses. This is certainly a far cry from the traditional skills attributed to health care managers.

Each of these developments can be traced back to a common origin; the advent of prospective payment as a vehicle for controlling soaring health care costs. Each brought with it a time of frenzied learning, in which health care managers were at first awestruck by the promise of the technologies of competition. With the emergence of each new force in health care management, though, managers feverishly mastered basic competencies in the disciplines, and came to understand them not as saviors of the health care industry but as competitive tools. That industry managers, most of whom had only scant if any formal training in these competencies, could so quickly come up to speed in competitive business management, speaks to both an industry imperative and the determination of health care managers to succeed.

Sophisticated Marketing

How did health care so quickly come to embrace the art and science of marketing as a tool to be used in management? The major impact of capitated reimbursement has been to reduce the amount of money received for treating any given patient malady. By limiting this payment per case, payors effectively forced providers to find ways to reduce the average length of stay (LOS) for patients. This means that the average LOS for treating pneumonia was reduced from perhaps seven to four days. At first, there was not much a hospital could do with an empty bed for three days, except hope to fill it with another patient. In order to get other patients, it became necessary to attract them from other places and convince them to use a specific hospital. But why should people change the hospital they use?

Enter marketing, with its research, demographic profiling, public relations strategy, and sophisticated use of advertising. In short order, professional marketing science enabled CEOs to understand how to attract patients and referring physicians, which zip-codes in a community were inhabited by people who both needed health care and could afford to pay for it, and what types of health care services were in greatest demand in the community. By its very nature, marketing requires tremendous amounts of detailed data about customer populations and their needs. In health care, "customer populations" is taken to mean patients who require health care services and their family members and physicians and institutions who make the determination of where a patient will receive needed health care.

In health care there is no one better positioned to provide such detailed information and monitor changes in customer needs and attitudes than the midlevel manager. It is this person who is in closest contact with all of the provider's customers, including patients, their families, physicians, and referring institutions. By virtue of this close contact with customers, the midlevel manager also has the potential to be a powerful "ambassador for the institution."

By using marketing as a competitive planning tool, managers have been able to develop services that were never before available in health care and offer them to the community almost overnight. These services are myriad and include such diverse areas as adult day care, child care, and clinics that specialize in providing routine care for working women, with office hours until 9:00 P.M. These services have increased in profitability in spite of reduced inpatient census population through the development of comprehensive market strategies that emphasize outpatient services and home care. They have enabled the development of joint ventures with key physicians in order to generate revenue and to provide those physicians with financial incentive to provide patient referrals.

How does the "average" health care manager use marketing as a competitive tool? She has become a front-line marketing generalist. Today's health care manager must assess the needs and wants of her customers and determine how well her staff and existing service structure are meeting those needs. She must also look into the crystal ball of market research and determine how those needs and wants will change over time. She must do this in order to anticipate those needs and to develop the services and staff to meet those needs before competing providers. Indeed, the health care manager is the marketing muscle for the provider. The successful manager does not wait for "marketing to tell us what we need to do." She uses the provider's marketing professionals as consultants to help her determine how best to assess customer trends and what factors will change in the community that will affect her department's services and staff. The role of the manager in the marketing-conscious world of health care is to use marketing to help monitor and interpret customer information in planning services and staffing to meet constantly changing community health needs. The manager in this role will use "corporate marketing" as advisers to help determine which information is most useful, how to best obtain that information, and what that information means to the organization as a whole.

It is the manager who must also determine what marketing intelligence means for her department. How does it affect the services available? Does she need to change the services available? Do the hours services are offered need to be changed? Are other hospitals providing the services available through the manager's department? If so, why should physicians and patients use this particular provider? What does the manager's department do that makes it different and more attractive to physicians and patients? How does the information impact her staffing practices? Does she need to change her staffing levels? Are her people providing a level of personal service to the patients and their families that will demonstrate true commitment and communicate a message of top-quality care? Only the manager is in a position to assess these and other very important questions raised by solid market information. The manager is the only individual in the entire organization who completely understands the talents and capacity of her department and the customer (that is, patients, physicians, families, and the community) well enough to be truly creative in assessing market opportunities to be tapped.

In one midwestern hospital I know, this critical role of the manager was very powerfully demonstrated. The director of dietary services in this hospital was faced with the dilemma of what to do with excess production and staffing capacity that had resulted from a chronic drop in patient census. Faced with an inability to purchase new, state-of-the-art food handling equipment and the very real possibility of staff layoffs in his area, the director took stock of his staff's talent and capacity and the hospital's stated desire to diversify services to new community segments and came up with a plan that might seem outlandish to many providers. Yet the idea proved extremely successful as a business venture and invaluable as a public relations effort for the hospital. The hospital began a catering business, providing all food for functions in two local hotels and donating services to local charities. With the added revenue from successful catering management, the director not only realized his goals but also extended the reach of the hospital into the daily lives of the community.

The lesson of this example? Only a manager who intimately knew the potential of the dietary services department could have and would have dared risk proposing such a concept. No one at a "corporate administration" level would be in a position to develop such a creative and successful way to turn a cost center into a revenue-generating center for the hospital.

To fulfill this creative potential, the director of dietary services had to redefine who he served. His customer was not just the patient and the cafeteria customer but also the community he served. A similar challenge faces all health care managers and has resulted in the emergence of the concept of the health care customer. While patients are still and will always be the reason for providing health care, managers now must consider not only the medical needs of the patient but also the customer service needs of the patient, the patient's family, and the people responsible for bringing the patient to any particular provider — the physicians. It is the manager's role to determine what these needs are and to instill in her staff a desire to address these customer service needs in every aspect of their work. To understand the reason for this, you need only answer one question. If two providers offer the same service — delivering a baby, perhaps — what determines which hospital an expectant mother, father, and their obstetrician will select? (Let's assume that the baby is not at risk and therefore is not expected to require special services.) The quality of care? In the traditional sense of "quality of care," probably not. Most patients have no idea about what really determines the medical quality of care; therefore, they will not make their choice based on that issue. While physicians certainly are in a position to evaluate this, it is unlikely that the quality of medicine practiced at hospital A is significantly better or worse than that practiced in hospital B in the same community. What is left then to influence the choice? Three things: price, convenience, and personal service. In my example of the food services director who dared to explore the possibilities within his grasp, he fulfilled the promise (indeed, obligation) of the midlevel manager and had a profound effect upon the organization as a whole. By catering to the community's dining public, he generated tremendous public regard for the hospital's ability to care for the area's personal service needs. With each successful function, the manager in effect generated positive publicity for the hospital.

Today's health care manager likely received little if any formal preparation in marketing or customer service. She may be uncomfortable with this new role. There is a choice for the manager. She can lead in exploiting market information, using marketing personnel as consultants and technical advisers to develop a dynamic and successful strategy. Or she can follow the lead of her counterparts in other hospitals who are exploiting the art and science of marketing. The rewards for leadership are greater now than ever before in the industry. The price of being a follower in a competitive health care environment is also great, for the manager and the organization.

Sophistication of Financial Management

Paralleling the development of sophisticated systems of marketing for provider services has been a maturing of the financial management system. Planning and controlling the financial strength of health care providers has changed more dramatically in the past few years than ever before in the history of the industry. The role of the midlevel manager in health care finance has grown along with the sophistication of the process.

Successful financial management once hinged on reimbursement based on cost-plus, investment income, and an active foundation office. Major development efforts were further supported with the issuance of debt. What changes have occurred in health care financial management to alter this strategy, and how has it been altered?

Impending revenue reductions as a result of capitated reimbursement, combined with continuous increases in the cost of supplies, have severely stressed the cash positions of many providers. This has led to the development of sophisticated and sometimes painful techniques for cost control throughout many organizations, with the department-level manager crucial to the success of these efforts. Examples of these efforts include inventory control systems; conversion of fixed costs, such as staff payroll, to variable cost elements, which could be increased or decreased as patient demand required; and permanent reductions in staff. To make these efforts work, chief administrators (who had now become CEOs) and chief financial officers relied heavily upon individual department managers to reduce operating costs within their limited scope of control. This grass-roots approach was and is necessary for the same reason that successful marketing efforts rely upon midlevel managers. That is where the most intimate knowledge of the process and people rests.

Other developments in the financial management of health care providers include the emergence of financial feasibility analysis applied to the strategic plan of the provider and to any proposed changes to a hospital's service line. Fiscal feasibility was once only a conceptual concern for health care managers. Managers recognized the need to be fiscally responsible, but were willing to undertake many projects and services, knowing full well that they would lose money. This risk was felt to be an acceptable cost of meeting the community's total health care wants and needs. Severe curtailment of available funding for such comprehensive services, however, meant that health care managers had to be more selective in developing services for community health needs. By and large, managers could only consider offering those services that would provide a stream of revenue with which to continue operation of the hospital.

Many new developments in financial management will continue to be introduced to the profession of health care management. Computer programs are being developed to model and analyze the financial performance of new service lines and of an entire organization under alternative scenarios. These models allow senior managers to predict, with reasonable accuracy, which investments will provide the greatest return for future financial health. Sophisticated systems of strategic capital planning, used in the rarified air of the CEO's office, allow executives far greater accuracy and effectiveness in planning the long-term ability of the organization to fund new health care services for the community. These subjects are treated thoroughly elsewhere (Kaufman and Hall, 1987), and the successful manager who wishes to continue that success is encouraged to explore these readings.

My purpose here is to explore the role of the manager in this changing financial environment. What do such abstract matters of return on investment, bond ratings, and debt to equity ratios have to do with managing a pediatrics center? Everything and more is the answer. One frustration common to all managers in health care is the chronic inability to offer all of the latest advances in care technology in the service-line of the hospital. Mastery of the concepts and, more importantly, the attitudes of fiscally responsible management will allow the manager to critically evaluate constantly evolving technologies and select from among them those offering the greatest promise for her customers and her department.

As an example of the importance of awareness of financial planning and management, consider the story of a manager who was responsible for the management of outpatient surgery at a large metropolitan hospital.

As director for the single freestanding outpatient surgery center run by his hospital, he was concerned with a trend that showed decreasing use of services for four months in a row. The problem, he knew, was largely one of location. The center was not in an area convenient to the homes of many potential customers; it was downtown, a few blocks away from the main campus of the hospital. Compounding this problem, a small group of surgeons, unaffiliated with the hospital, had opened two competing centers, and both were nearer to the community of potential patients.

Realizing that the cost of moving the one center to an area with two competing centers was great, the manager explored other avenues of recapturing lost patient volume. He conducted his own financial analysis of his competition and studied their strengths and weaknesses carefully. While it was true that the competing centers had begun to gather a regular flow of pa-tients and referrals, they did have potential problems that might be unseen by a manager unconcerned with the finances of competition.

Estimating the cost of managing a center, the inconve-nience of not having a strong hospital affiliation (as his com-petitors did not), and other operating expenses including heavy costs for professional liability, diagnostic service contracts, and facility maintenance, the manager concluded that his com-petitors might be happier as his customers, or as partners with his hospital in providing outpatient surgical care. The idea the manager proposed to his vice president was ultimately modified to accommodate new and more comprehensive information about the market, true costs, and the financial position of the competing surgical group. What resulted from the initiative of a single manager, however, was an agreement that allowed the hospital to lease and manage both of the competing centers, in return for staff privileges and shared profits in all three centers for the partners of the private surgical group. In essence, the manager initiated a joint venture with an external concern that provided important services to the community and improved the hospital's financial position.

Community Market Segmentation

The financial feasibility of health care services, combined with a new understanding of the marketplace, also influenced health care managers to alter the fundamental mission of the organization. No longer could every provider be a full-service organization, dedicated to meeting the total needs of every resident in the community. Some providers focus upon the needs of the family, while others emphasize services for the elderly or other segments of the community. In short, managers began to focus on serving the total needs of a smaller section of the community and allowing other providers to develop comprehensive services for other groups.

The trend toward market segmentation has certain potential advantages for the manager who strives to provide the best care possible for his customers. He can devote more time and energy to completely and creatively developing services tailored to the medical and customer service needs of smaller market segments. This market segmentation has brought about the conveniences offered by adult day-care centers and family centered birthing suites.

The same trend, however, also creates a concern for health care managers and for the community: If market segmentation and service development are determined by financial feasibility, will the less lucrative but equally important segments of the community be neglected by providers? Will public hospitals be forced to provide care for an increasingly large number of people who are unable to pay for that care, because those people have been refused care at private hospitals? Chicago's Cook County Hospital, a public institution, regularly admits patients without any insurance or ability to pay for health care. Many of these patients have already been to two other area providers and been refused care. This "patient dumping," selectively admitting only patients with documentable ability to pay, puts the rejected patients at increased risk. It also places a legal, moral, and financial burden upon municipal hospitals that are typically the recipients of dumped patients.

The answer to the threat posed by such dumping is still evolving and a matter of considerable debate. In some communities, it is a matter left to the provider institutions and charitable organizations to resolve. In others, legislation has been adopted to curb this unethical segmentation of the patient care marketplace. Enforcement of these well-intentioned laws, how-ever, has been a challenge because of the difficulty of proving patient dumping. In the final analysis, it will be the health care manager who answers this question, either by neglecting un-profitable segments of the community health care market or by finding innovative ways to manage their health care to make them profitable.

Decentralization of Delivery Systems

Market segmentation, customer service orientation, and the promise of reduced operating costs have also led to the transformation of the delivery system used to provide health care to the community. While once the hospital was the only place patients could receive medical care, it is now only used when more convenient and less costly vehicles are unavailable. Examples of more convenient, less costly delivery vehicles in-clude freestanding outpatient surgery and urgent care centers, mobile laboratories and radiology centers, and home health care. Some hospitals and physician groups are even experiment-ing with the resurrection of the physician who makes house calls! Each of these services provides medical care that was previously available only in the hospital.

As the industry moves forward, the structure of this de-centralized network of care delivery will certainly change as managers discover new ways to harness technology for health care. Computers will enable remote site managers to instantly transfer and receive administrative and clinical information between sites. Artificial intelligence systems will allow clinicians at satellite centers to develop accurate diagnoses and treatment regimes without the benefit of the physical presence of spe-cialists. Soft technologies of human performance improvement and sociotechnical engineering will enable satellite center staff to function more efficiently than ever before, even though they are isolated from the resources of parent organizations. While the exact form of the satellite center of tomorrow is yet to evolve, one thing is certain: It will evolve and play an ever-increasing role in the delivery of health care. The successful health care manager of tomorrow must develop the skills needed to master the challenges presented by this new force in health care.

The certainty of continued decentralization presents a host of new challenges to all health care managers, from clinical supervisors to the CEO. How do you project service utilization and staffing patterns in a new center? How do you efficiently manage communications and quality assurance? What kind of decision-making authority will have to be delegated to care givers in a clinic that may be miles away from the parent institution? How do you monitor staff performance and customer satisfaction from a distance? Even issues as mundane as equipment delivery and maintenance become added concerns for managers. In this era of networked medicine, the planning, control, and human resource functions of health care management become not merely important but crucial to the success of care delivery.

Consumerism in Health Care

Until recently, the opinion of the care giver was sacred. Patients and families did not question the wisdom of a physician's decision. This has begun to change and will continue to do so to a much greater degree. Patients are beginning to insist upon having a voice as a partner in the planning of their care, and this presents both challenge and opportunity for clinicians and managers alike.

Why this emerging consumerism in health care, and how does it affect the manager? There are two important reasons for the development of consumerism in health care. The first is a rising level of public knowledge about health care choices and the potential for harmful side effects as well as for curative effects of any particular treatment regime. As the public becomes more informed, there is increased need and demand for a greater role in the planning of care.

The second major cause of consumerism is a steadily growing portion of health care payments that comes directly from the pocket of the consumer. Insurance coverage provided by employers is the single most common source of payment for health care in the country. Over the past fifteen years, this insurance has changed from a system of first-dollar payment at 80 to 100 percent of incurred costs to one in which the employee must share the burden for payment on a sliding scale. This means that in matters of routine illness, where costs are (relatively) lower, the patient is paying for a larger portion of the care. With this financial incentive, the patient and his family find the prospect of questioning medical decisions and seeking second opinions less intimidating than paying perhaps several hundred dollars for an initially recommended care plan.

How does this affect the manager? She will find herself on the receiving end of questions about not only the efficacy of services rendered but also the cost of line items on patient bills after discharge. She will be challenged to demonstrate the achievement of the highest possible quality services at the lowest possible prices. Where costs are higher, the health care manager will be held accountable to demonstrate a significant improvement in value of services that more than justify that higher price tag. The manager will have to become an educator, providing the public with the knowledge needed to make intelligent decisions about their health care. Finally, the manager will serve as the primary consumer communication conduit for the organization. In this role the manager will educate the provider about the needs and attitudes of the community using her department's services.

How will the health care manager anticipate and manage the challenge of consumerism? In addition to financial and marketing skills, the manager must effectively tap the talent of his staff through effective supervision of people and through development of that staff. Successful management of people and education and training with value for the individual and the provider organization are the keys to handling the demands of consumerism. As I will show in later chapters, these two tools are also critical for other areas of health care management. For now, though, let us focus on the roles they will play in managing consumerism.

Effective people management enables the manager to select and develop a staff who are sensitive to and knowledgeable about consumers' need for knowledge. It also allows the manager to use each staff member as an information source providing ongoing feedback about consumers. These same skills will empower the manager to effectively work with the community to address consumer concerns directly and cooperatively and create allies in the community. People management skills and a commitment to consumers' right to know were responsible for Johnson & Johnson's effective handling of a nationwide crisis in consumer confidence. This crisis occurred when the product Tylenol was poisoned not once, but twice. By effectively demonstrating concern for consumer fears and providing information directly and quickly to those consumers, the company not only prevented problems but actually strengthened customer commitment.

The use of education and training to manage consumerism means that a manager accepts personal responsibility for the education of two groups of people about critical aspects of his services. The manager must assess and meet the knowledge needs of the consumer and of his staff.

Community education about health care traditionally focuses on ways to avoid disease and on ways to manage the care of chronic conditions such as cardiopulmonary disease or Alzheimer's disease. Many aggressive managers, however, are expanding upon this and are using education as a way to enlighten the public about how to evaluate the quality of medical care offered and how to become effective consumers of health care. In doing this, these managers are creating a trust with the community and are fulfilling an essential human need: the need to understand. Examples of this include sports-medicine clinics that offer free or inexpensive educational programs on evaluating sports-medicine support centers and managing injuries, as well as educational symposia sponsored by hospitals for another segment of the consumer market, physicians and allied health professionals.

Staff education requires that the manager focus upon the skill and knowledge needs of his staff. These skills and areas of knowledge are also different from those provided in traditional in-service education settings. The skills needed by the staff to

make them individual agents of consumer education and customer relations span beyond the boundaries of clinical theory
and practice. These skills encompass effective interpersonal
communication and selling concepts and a fundamental knowledge of medical economics as it affects the department. Staff
training must be managed to address the skill and knowledge
necessary for the real world that is not covered in medical or
allied health professional curricula.

Overall Impact of Trends

How have these trends permanently altered health care as
an industry? The industry has become tremendously more sophisticated as it has assumed responsibility for its own fiscal
destiny. The provider of the early 1970s did not have organized
efforts at strategic planning, market research and development,
product (service) line management, physician joint ventures, or
satellite business development. Health care public relations was
prehistoric by the standards of twentieth-century business management, and the thought of paying for and measuring the
impact of advertising was unheard of. Customer service was not
even a phrase heard in the hospital corridors twenty years ago,
let alone the battle cry of entire organizations that it has become. Today, these things are commonplace, and organizations
without these tools have long since become unprofitable and
were forced to close or merge with other providers that were in a
more solid fiscal position. This trend will continue, and health
care will become a competitive profit-oriented industry exploiting all of the same business management technologies that have
long been used by the Fortune 500. The challenge facing the
industry is twofold. It must continue on its course of accelerated
learning and master the business management skills of the
twenty-first century, and it must find solutions to the moral and
ethical dilemma of providing care to the financially disen-
franchised of the community. In short, the industry must become shrewd at the business of business and not lose its commitment to humanity.

These trends require the manager to learn more each

week about business decision making. But the greatest challenge facing the manager is to her skills in handling people's performance. Virtually every major industry trend to date has had enormous ramifications for the management of people in the provider organization. In 1986–1987, a survey conducted for the American College of Healthcare Executives (Stevens, 1987b) sought to determine the most pressing issues regarding people's performance. A sample of nearly 200 CEOs, chief financial officers, and other top executives identified two factors that they feel will have a long-term impact on staff performance levels: (1) constantly changing technologies in both health care science and business management that demand more rapid acquisition of skills and (2) a need to change the way *all* personnel view their work as professionals in the delivery of health care. The senior managers surveyed clearly expressed the importance of each person becoming more intimately involved in the business of health care, while not for a minute reducing their commitment to quality patient care. This change will result in staff who are entrepreneurial in their approach to doing even daily work and are able to experiment with new ways to provide care and with developing new services for the community. This need to change the way people approach their work in health care is the result of a failure of people in health care to adapt their performance to the demands of a changing work environment. In recognizing this, executives in organizations around the nation have begun to lead a grass-roots commitment to business creativity and individual responsibility in health care and other industries. Without this commitment to the business issues of health care delivery, there will be no way to pay for health care. Or, put succinctly, "No margin—no mission."

How exactly does the manager become business savvy and entrepreneurial, much less develop a staff like that? To do this the health care manager must radically realign how he views his role and his business. This paradigm shift in the way one views the manager's role will change nothing about the manager's responsibility in the hospital. It will change, however, the things that occupy a manager's time to fulfill that responsibility. To help managers make this shift in how they view their work, we must

examine briefly the ideal role of an effective health care manager and then compare that role to some commonly held beliefs
about the manager's job.

The health care manager's entire purpose is simply to
enable. The manager enables his people to provide their services
in the most effective way possible both to serve the patient (and
internal clients) and to provide some return to the provider
organization. The manager is no longer solely a technical expert. For example, while the director of nursing likely possesses
extremely competent clinical skills, her job is not to nurse. It is to
make certain that clinical nurses have the support, direction,
and resources to nurse. Thus, while the director is a nurse by
training and certainly in heart, her professional commitment is
no longer to nurse. She is a manager of people's performance
and is evaluated as such by the CEO or associate administrator
to whom she reports.

Myths of Health Care Management

The many prevalent myths about the management of
people, common among professional managers, prevent many
health care managers from realizing the potential of one who
enables performance. Let us examine a few of the more prevalent myths that stand between health care managers and the
successful assumption of this broader leadership role.

> *Management Myth 1:* The role of management is pri-
> marily to plan, staff, acquire resources, implement ser-
> vices, and evaluate the success of a department.

This managerial role can be found in every classic text on
management, regardless of the industry being managed. My
particular description is a paraphrase from the Catholic Hospital Press texts on health care management. This "classic" definition may have applied in some bygone era for health care, but it
is inadequate for the contemporary age of medicine. This definition focuses on the need for the manager to Control with a
capital "C" the operations of his people and department. Con-

trol, however, is a counterproductive concept for managers. It implies, in theory and often in practice, the restraint and containment of operations and people. Today's health care manager cannot succeed by trying vainly to control his department. Such a manager may as well try to tie a leash around an elephant, forcing it to follow only a narrow, set path. We can easily surmise what will happen to someone who spends any time at the back end of an elephant. The manager's staff behind him and the manager himself cannot control the beast in between them (the organization). Changes in conditions and priorities for the "beast" may create a mess for those leading the control (the manager) and those following behind.

The managerial function that must replace control is the leadership and creative use of the department's capital and human resources in the service of organizational goals. The manager who abandons control in favor of guidance and leadership would sit atop an elephant and guide it to a destination. This manager will allow the power of the elephant to influence the exact path of travel, while occasionally nudging it to ensure that its overall direction is toward important goals. Why let the elephant influence the precise path followed? It has the best understanding of its power and the clearest perspective of the easiest path to follow.

Peter Drucker (1989) once observed that the American management model is based upon a structure that was successful for a time in the manufacturing segment of industry. In a bygone era of industrial youth, the management functions of all American businesses, including health care, were modeled after manufacturing giants of the nation. In this era, we turned to General Motors and to Chrysler to find management role models. In these plants, and thirty years ago, this myth may have been reality. Today, however, health care is at once blessed and cursed by a marketplace more dynamic than any ever faced by automotive or service industries. Another difference between health care and the classic industry model is its work force. Health care workers are not the skilled tradesmen and unskilled labor of the auto manufacturing industry and cannot be managed as if they were. The health care work force in today's community hospital is composed almost exclusively of well-educated professionals who work willingly for mediocre salaries. This health care work force is very diverse in all but two characteristics: a solid academic background and staunch professionalism. The manager's role in this environment is not to obsess about the control of a repetitive process but to empower autonomous professionals to continually improve upon what they see as their humanitarian mission. This real-life role of the health care manager is far more exciting and important than the mythical one.

Management Myth 2:   Staff training and development are the primary responsibility of corporate offices of continuing education and organization development.

In an institution as complex and diverse as the health care provider organization, it is impossible to understand the precise needs of individual departments from a corporate office. Indeed, the only person who can provide the necessary mix of objective business analysis and professional technical knowledge is the department manager. It is a rare staff person in a department who can provide the business perspective needed to plan training and development that will focus on the business and market priorities of the organization, in addition to the skills of his or her profession. Corporate offices of education and organization development are similarly handicapped with respect to the unique needs of a single department. These offices can, however, be resources to the manager who would direct training. They can support the manager in determining needs and in finding training resources to best meet the needs specified by the manager. Within the limits of their technical expertise, each of these offices can also provide faculty and training design assistance for specific programs. Offices of education and organization development can be consultants to and resources for the line manager. Only that line manager has the appropriate business perspective and technical knowledge to direct the training needs of her staff. In this way, the manager's relationship with training and organization development is sim-

Figure 1.1. Components of Performance.

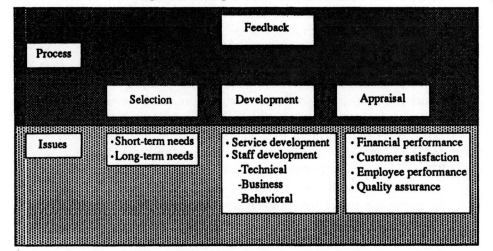

ilar to her relationship with the marketing department, as was discussed earlier.

> *Management Myth 3*: The major benefit of employee development is to the employee who becomes a more marketable quantity and is paid by the employer for doing so.

In any employee development experience, there is gain to the employee. If properly planned and guided by the manager, though, there is also demonstrable payback to the organization as well. Conversely, if employee development is not managed wisely to meet the needs of both employer and employee, the employee may or may not receive significant dividends on the company's investment, and the company will undoubtedly receive little added value. In the end, if employee development is given little or no concerted management-level guidance, both parties will surely pay a price in performance.

A New Focus in Health Care Management

Industry leaders believe that the manager's responsibility for supervising people is critical to success. I agree with these leaders. But what exactly is performance management? And if managers spend all of their time managing this, how will they oversee such priorities as a budget, quality control, and work flow? Let us look at what must be done to manage people's performance.

Directing a staff in health care means focusing on four key processes: systematic staff selection, ongoing staff development integrated with the business plans of the organization, continuous (rather than annual) performance appraisal, and constant feedback to staff on the effectiveness of their performance. There is usually something that passes for these processes in most businesses. But these components of performance management are rarely undertaken by managers (health care or otherwise) with the same analytical rigor as, say, the components of financial management. Let us look at the components in Figure 1.1 and see how they affect performance management in health care. The relationship among these four components is similar to that of organ systems in the study of medicine. In medicine, each organ system, such as the circulatory system, has its own purpose. It must be managed as an individual entity. Yet each is also dependent on other systems, such as the respiratory and the nervous systems, to survive. Similarly, to conduct training and development in a manner to achieve peak staff performance, the health care manager must understand how the system works with interdependent systems. A brief look at the interaction among the "organ systems" of staff performance follows.

The Selection System

A manager needs a personnel selection system to recruit and screen qualified employees. There are three important points to make about the selection system with regard to the line manager in health care and training and development.

> *Selection Point 1*: An effective selection system must screen potential employees to determine not only tech-

nical competence but interpersonal and attitudinal characteristics as well.

In one hospital, a colleague of mine spent much of his time for nearly a year as a referee of frequent and serious disputes between a brilliant young nurse and equally competent, but much more seasoned nurses. In many of these disputes, which occurred frequently in the most inappropriate of places, such as the Intensive Care Unit, the primary cause was an inappropriate level of aggressiveness and a simply offensive style of communication on the part of the young nurse. In one case, physically separating combatants was required. Use of a selection system that addressed these critical survival skills for the hospital floor would have been very useful to this manager when interviewing the young nurse prior to employment.

> *Selection Point 2*: The quality of a selection system in a hospital can affect training and development efforts in a manager's area. Less obvious is the impact that training quality has on the effectiveness of a selection system.

This point is clearly shown in a case recorded by Burke in 1978. In this case, a newly hired director of nursing (DON), after assessing her nursing staff, determined that staffing levels were inadequate, and 40 percent of the existing staff was functionally incompetent. The DON established an effective selection system to ensure that only competent nurses would be hired in the future. Only after recruiting efforts were an abysmal failure did the DON learn that her new employer had a reputation for being a "leper colony" of professional development. Virtually no quality training and development was conducted in the hospital. As a result, competent nurses had no interest in working at that hospital. The DON learned very painfully that inadequate training crippled a sound selection system and reduced managerial ability to improve people performance.

> *Selection Point 3*: Managers often fail to use a selection system well, if at all.

The best explanation I have heard for this phenomenon was at a recent conference, where a keynote speaker observed, "The reason managers have such a terrible track record at selecting high performers is that they think it's a matter of common sense. They figure that anybody with half a brain can spot talent." As a result, managers look only for one or two critical indicators of talent, usually in the area of technical expertise. In a hospital, however, only 20 percent of the performance problems result from problems with technical ability. Eighty percent of the performance headaches the typical manager faces are caused by other domains of performance. A system of selection can address these areas more accurately than "common sense"— if that system accurately assesses both quantitative and qualitative traits of candidates.

The Development System

A system of development includes continuing education, ongoing coaching, and untraditional learning experiences such as mentorship programs and special project assignments. Performance managers use these development experiences in unique combinations for each employee. The goal of the development system is to match precisely for each employee only those experiences that will correct skill deficits or provide new skills that are important to both the business goals of the department and the personal goals of the employee. The tool a manager uses in this process is a negotiated development contract, which matches specific experiences to expected dates of completion and, where possible, specifies expected performance changes that will occur as a result of development. This development contract then becomes a focus of ongoing assessment and performance appraisal.

> *Development Point 1*: The performance benefit of employee development for the health care provider is often not realized because development is not planned and managed in a systematic fashion.

When a new employee is hired, it is assumed that she has all of the skills necessary to perform effectively at a specific job. Orientation is often provided about personnel rules and regulations, available benefits, and the existence of an evil underground empire, the labor union. In technical positions (in health care that covers most positions), some further orientation may be given about a particular infusion system, lab equipment, or refrigeration system. From this point, employee development often has four components:

- In-service education to review medical topics or explore new technology being used by the provider
- Monthly/annual professional symposia, which serve as the *USA Today* of professional development, covering everything under the sun and all of it superficially
- Behavioral skill development (maybe), which takes place in either a three-day marathon session or a two-hour *Reader's Digest* condensed version
- Voluntary participation in formal degree programs through local colleges, using an employer-funded tuition reimbursement program

Such development methods are useful but inadequate if development is expected to improve job performance. None of them will change employees' performance appreciably without the addition of managerial involvement to make certain that skills are needed, coached, and used on the job. The manager can ensure this by using many strategies, but the strategies must be ongoing and focused on using employee development contracts.

The Assessment System

The third determinant of performance is the assessment system in place in a hospital. The sum of all tools used to measure performance, the assessment system includes financial assessment, quality assurance, and management evaluation systems in addition to staff performance assessment. Typically, we tend to consider each of these assessment functions separately, rather than as interrelated pieces of the total performance system for which the manager is responsible. Thus, we only consider financial performance on a monthly basis, when budget reports are produced, and in the last quarter of the fiscal year, when planning is under way. In doing this, we miss an opportunity to evaluate how performance in one area affects another area of performance. The purpose of the assessment system is to provide feedback about the effectiveness of the entire realm of the manager, not just people's performance or any single performance area.

When combined with information about financial and operational performance of a department, a review of performance appraisals of an entire department can provide a manager with much useful information when planning development for her staff. For example, the manager reviewing performance appraisals for her department might notice that several people have a common performance need, which might be met in part by management training of these people. In a true performance management system, the assessment system includes analysis of operational and financial performance indicators also, in order to assess the performance of staff in these areas. Here is a simple illustration of how these indicators can be used to directly manage people's performance. Reviewing operational and financial performance for the department might reveal excess spending for disposable equipment compared to patient charges for disposables. This might indicate several needs, including a training need for staff. This training might be in proper procedures for documenting disposable equipment used in caring for each patient.

> *Assessment Point 1*:   Assessment must be an ongoing process in order to shape, rather than simply to judge, people's performance.

Most organizations have a performance assessment system for personnel that includes employee evaluation after some initial period of probationary employment (ninety days or six months), and subsequent annual performance appraisals. These annual appraisals are often used essentially to determine the size of a merit raise. What typically happens in these systems goes something like this: A week before the evaluation is due, the manager pulls any previous assessments from an employee file, along with any performance notes that may (or may not) have been kept. Reviewing the appraisal form to reacquaint himself with assessment criteria, the manager then tries to recall over the span of a year specific instances in which the employee performed well or poorly in each performance area. To get corroboration, the manager may then ask for input from other supervisors or managers with whom the employee has worked. Then the manager reviews his assessment with the employee, a merit raise is determined from a fixed scale, and the employee returns to work—rarely ecstatic, often neutral, and sometimes feeling victimized by the process.

With this system, the employee is never apprised of performance needs at a time when she can do anything to improve them. If an employee has an altercation with a physician, manager, or peer in March that a manager observes and is then evaluated in December based upon this instance, which is particularly memorable to the manager, two things have likely occurred. The manager did not observe other situations from April until December showing the employee's ability to handle similar situations, and the manager may not have evaluated the cause of the performance problem and developed the employee's skill in the area. All that has occurred is the passing of judgment. Both the manager and the employee have missed an opportunity to improve performance. A manager of performance will use the assessment process in a structured, ongoing fashion both to improve the accuracy of annual performance appraisals and to constantly diagnose and boost the level of staff performance.

Feedback

Feedback is to performance management what the body's nervous system is to life. Just as the nervous system relays signals to the brain and endocrine systems about the status of the heart and lungs, so does management feedback provide both the manager and staff with the status of performance within a department. Because of this vital role, feedback should be only slightly less frequent than nerve impulse transmission. Feed-back about the effectiveness of staff performance must be fre-quent enough to allow staff to modify their performance as soon as necessary to improve patient care or operating efficiency. Monitoring performance for weeks or months and then present-ing a list of sorts to staff about where they fell short of expecta-tions will not improve performance. This approach to feedback is not timely and is certainly not specific enough to be of help in focusing on specific behaviors that can be improved. It will only provide them with a broadly focused critique of their performance.

Most health care managers would not disagree with this premise—at least not in theory. But in practical application, getting and giving adequate feedback can become overwhelm-ing, occupying so much of a manager's time that other impor-tant functions are neglected in pursuit of this goal. In the following chapters of this book, I will provide practical tools to help the manager establish a feedback network that taps all of the people and administrative systems of the organization to manage feedback. By using these other information sources as components of a system of feedback management, the manager can provide and receive this feedback in a timely manner with-out stretching herself so thin that professional burnout is a threat.

The Total Management System

How does a manager integrate these components of man-aging in the face of unprecedented change in the industry with the classic functions of management on a day-to-day basis? This really will not be a problem when you see that there is great overlap between the two approaches to managing. The skills necessary for this new management focus will also strengthen the traditional administrative functions already mastered by health care managers. These five classic administrative functions of management are:

- Planning
- Organizing
- Staffing
- Implementing
- Controlling operations

Many management texts address these functions from a macro perspective. That is, they treat these functions by describing the components of each function that must be addressed by a successful manager. What these traditional texts overlook, however, are the detailed activities of the process of managing these components. Let us examine how one manages these five functions and the importance of the skills employed in this process to proactive management.

> *Management Point 1*: Skills that are common to both effective management and powerful performance management are setting goals for staff performance, coaching, counseling, and team leadership.

If these skills are used well in the five classic functions of management, they will also catalyze performance management efforts. If they are not done well, they will at best not reinforce other effective practices.

> *Management Point 2*: These critical skills are the subject of most management seminars, and yet they are the same ones presenting the greatest ongoing challenge for most managers.

These behavioral skills, goal setting, coaching, counseling, and team leadership, form the core of successful management of an entrepreneurial staff—a staff that incorporates business savvy into their repertoire of regularly practiced professional skills. The manager who successfully uses these skills in the classic functions of management can apply them as well in her role as a manager of training and development.

Setting goals for staff performance is critical to the manager as it not only guides performance directly but it also flags areas of need for further training and helps to reinforce learning that occurs in the training class. As I will demonstrate in Chapter Seven, explicit performance goal setting is crucial to the success of training staff.

The manager who coaches staff on the clinical floor on a regular basis is helping her staff transfer the use of newly learned and seldom used skills to routine use in daily job performance. This single management role is the biggest difference between training that stays in the classroom and training that comes alive in the workplace. As a coach, the manager must also practice the art of "managing by wandering around," to reinforce in staff an understanding of the business ramifications of their behavior. This is especially true with medical and allied health staffs, where many years of training and service in the humanitarian art of healing often create a condescending opinion of the "crass" nature of business and fiscal responsibility. The manager must show his staff through the coaching process that intelligent, entrepreneurial management is not the same as "placing a dollar value on human life," as many medical professionals believe. In fact, in today's health care arena, often only entrepreneurial approaches to business enable the development of new humanitarian services for community health. Managers coach their staff in many areas of job performance on a daily basis. Observing staff performance and providing feedback to improve that performance is a primary way that staff develop clinical, supervisory, and interpersonal communication skills. This same process can be used to develop staff ability to think about and evaluate individual and department performance from an entrepreneurial perspective as well.

Supportive rather than judgmental management counseling is often the only way a staff person can pinpoint the cause and solutions to personal performance problems. These same skills are an integral part of the training functions of practice, feedback, and evaluation. In this way, counseling is a skill both the manager and the trainer use to improve staff competence.

Dynamic team leadership by a manager is the key to organizing, overcoming individual differences, and working co-operatively in a health care setting. Team leadership in today's hospital is even more essential than in the hospital of ten years ago. This is easily demonstrated by emerging medical technolo-gies. Successful use of technology to provide total heart-lung support, for example, is only possible with interdisciplinary teamwork from physicians, nurses, and at least a half-dozen other allied health professions. Without strong team leadership from managers, training in the myriad sciences necessary for interdisciplinary health care would have little if any positive impact on the delivery of emerging therapies.

The determinants of peak staff performance are also in the realm of "classic" management. No one would argue that staff selection, performance assessment, and day-to-day management are not the responsibility of the traditional health care manager. Yet, as we have seen, each of these skills is also inextricably linked with effective management of people in times of rapid and unpredictable change. If the skills are used effectively in both areas of responsibility, management effectiveness with each will enhance the performance of the other. The remainder of this book addresses practical strategies that enable managers to achieve excellence in the quality of service provided by their departments in the constantly changing, competitive environ-ment of modern health care delivery.

2

Responsive Leadership:
Key Roles and
Responsibilities

Harold Geneen, former CEO of ITT, said of leadership that "it cannot be taught. It can only be learned." This captain of industry went on to liken leadership to the sport of baseball. Just as no great ball player ever learned to field or to hit a home run by reading a book, Geneen contends that no great leader acquired that ability from a text. The purpose of this chapter is not to teach a health care manager how to lead. Its purpose is, however, to provide direction about what leaders have in common and what differentiates a manager-leader from a manager. This chapter will present six responsibilities of leadership in a department, describe how those responsibilities are met successfully, and provide an opportunity to evaluate your approach to leadership.

Why be a leader? The question may seem unnecessary at first. It is akin to asking "Why be intelligent?" or "Why be successful?" These are all desirable attributes to many people. The answer, though, for health care managers is tremendously important. First, the very role of the manager carries with it leadership responsibility. This is characteristic of every industry and will not be belabored. Second, in any time of rapid and unpredictable change, leadership provides the vision, specific direction, and stability necessary to enable progress and success. And nowhere, except perhaps Eastern Europe, is there more rapid and confusing change than in health care. Some of these changes were outlined in Chapter One, but that was a brief synopsis. While not every leader is a manager, in health care, every great manager must first be a leader.

Characteristics and Responsibilities of Leadership

The literal definition of a leader is "to guide or direct on a course or in a direction." While this definition is succinct and in essence accurate, it does little to help us understand what a leader must be. By this literal definition, a dictator qualifies as a leader and yet would certainly be ineffective as a health care leader.

Of more help is an understanding of the *responsibilities* of a leader and the demonstrable *outcomes* of effective leadership. Effective leadership has many different styles, depending on the leader and organizational culture. But all effective leaders are committed to fulfilling six different responsibilities. After describing each of these responsibilities briefly, I will present challenges associated with each of them.

1. *Be the source of a vision* that will guide staff as they manage in both stable and changing environments. In an environment as dynamic as health care, this responsibility is crucial. A manager's vision in times of change serves the same purpose as a sailor's sextant during a storm. That purpose is to guide the direction of effort toward a goal when shifting weather obscures the way.
2. *Establish and maintain trust.* This trust is reflected in the everyday management activities of the leader, as well as during times of significant change. The leader is responsible for maintaining the trust of his subordinates and for maintaining trust between his superiors and peers in management as well. A high level of trust is often demonstrated in departments where problems are quickly identified and resolved and where innovation is attempted regularly. A lack of trust, on the other hand, at the very least will slow

progress in a department and at its worst will destroy the staff's ability to function as a team.

3. *Serve as political conduit* between the department and the organization. To contribute to the success of both the department and the provider, the manager must lead the department in the political arena that is bounded by senior administration, the medical staff, and other departments. While trust is a prerequisite to effective political leadership, many other factors determine a manager's success in the political realm of an organization. Among these factors are knowledge of cultural norms and taboos in the organization, awareness and intelligent use of the formal and informal power structure in the provider, and effective monitoring of changes in these areas. In her role as political conduit, the manager ensures that important initiatives of the department are given both political and resource support and that important department interests become important organizational interests.

4. *Serve as ethical standard-bearer for the department.* Effective leaders set and maintain standards of ethical conduct for their staff and frequently for others in the organization. In accepting this responsibility, leaders understand the burden of consistency and the power of the role model to influence behavior. The ethical leader understands and demonstrates the difference between what is ethically *wrong* and legally or culturally *accepted*, as well as the difference between what is ethically *correct*, but legally or culturally *unacceptable*. The manager demonstrates ethical leadership by weighing carefully each decision he makes and its potential benefit or risk against a clearly defined personal code of ethics. When there is a conflict between the decision or action and the code, the leader must act in concert with the code.

5. *Make decisions.* The manager-leader understands and accepts the role of decision maker. This responsibility can be shared, in consensus decision making, but even when doing this, the manager has decided to share the task of making a decision and to abide by that decision. While decision-

making styles of individuals may be very different, depending upon a given situation, the nature of the decision being
made, and the individual manager, the manager-leader
must still accept accountability for decisions affecting her
department.

6. *Judge.* Different from decision making, the leader's responsibility to serve as judge truly separates him from his subordinates and from superiors in administration. Subordinates
are subject to judgment, while superiors and peers cannot
undo a leader's judgment. In making a decision, a leader
may simply choose between alternatives. In passing judgment, often an uncomfortable responsibility, the leader
must determine the *value* of an employee, a policy, or other
element of the department's operations. Value is often affected by current department needs, but the bottom line is
acceptance or rejection. Effective leadership requires that
the manager understand the department's needs, her own
ethical position, and her own decision-making practices.
Too little judgment by a manager creates inertia in a department that is often embodied by ineffective staff continuing
in their positions or failure to change policy important for
growth. Too much or indiscriminate judgment by a manager creates an environment of fear and indecisiveness
among staff and uncertainty among peers and superiors.

These six responsibilities of leadership are not isolated
from each other. A manager's effectiveness at passing judgment
will be influenced by his ethical position, decision-making style,
and other facets of leadership. Similarly, a leader's political
effectiveness will be affected by the level of trust existing between her and others and the vision of success she communicates to and shares with others.

Leadership Styles

The style of leadership a manager exhibits is the result of
how he balances each of these six responsibilities. The actions a
leader demonstrates create for his staff, peers, and superiors a

composite portrait of his effectiveness and style of leadership. Often, others will not be able to explain precisely why they trust someone's ability to lead, particularly if that person does not fit the stereotypical American model of the bold, independent rogue leader romanticized in westerns and war movies. What they will say, however, is, "I trust him," or "She'll get the job done."

There are many different models of leadership; each attempts to define the critical determinants of success or at least explain failure at effective leadership. These models include Stogdill's Two-Dimensional Leadership Model (1974), Likert's System 4 Management Model (1976), and the Managerial Grid offered by Blake and Mouton (1988). These models are useful as conceptual frameworks and are highly recommended for reference and background information. Here, however, I will focus in general terms on leadership styles and then describe how a manager must fulfill the responsibilities of leadership in the health care environment.

The most effective style of leadership for any manager is determined by two factors:

1. *The individual*, who brings to her practice of leadership the habits, skills, and conscious or unconscious behaviors that affect her fulfillment of each of the six responsibilities of a leader. This "internal" facet of leadership is the result of the combined experiences of the individual. This experience can include childhood and adolescent socialization and formal training and education.
2. *The environment* or work situation in which the leader is functioning. Often, a particular leadership challenge or sudden change in a management environment will influence what is most effective for leading a department. For example, when faced with restructuring a department as a result of a merger or shift in services being offered, a manager might rely upon a participative style of leadership and seek consensus from his supervisors about alternatives and optimal choices. This has the advantage of supplying multiple perspectives and helps ensure cooperation with any future decisions related to the restructuring.

Figure 2.1. Responsive Leadership.

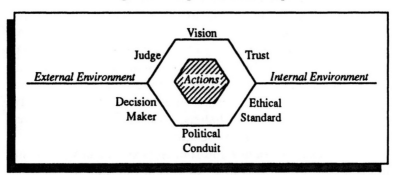

The effectiveness of a manager's leadership depends to a great extent upon his flexibility to meet his responsibilities as a leader using different approaches to solving problems and upon his ability to monitor and respond to environmental conditions. Some leadership challenges are best met with a participative style of management, and others are best managed with an autocratic approach.

In general then, the aggregate success of the manager-leader will depend on the manager's ability to apply a variety of management and leadership strategies and to assess and implement the most effective strategies for a given work environment. This does not mean that the manager has several leadership styles, but that his style is responsive to the needs of the people, politics, and business issues of his workplace.

Responsive Leadership

The responsive leader determines what her actions will be by balancing her own preferred style of managing the six major leadership responsibilities and the style required for optimal effectiveness given the organizational, environmental, and situational factors that influence effective decision making. The relationship is shown in Figure 2.1.

Responsive leadership is an ongoing process in which the manager fulfills six core responsibilities, balancing two forces that at times oppose each other and at times may be in concert with each other. The first of the forces balanced are the internal beliefs, convictions, and preferred approaches to managing each of the six responsibilities of leadership. This internal environment of leadership is what the manager brings to the organization. The second of these forces balanced by the responsive leader is the external environment, which includes organizational values and beliefs, time factors, interpersonal factors, and other situation-specific forces.

One example of how internal and external environments interact in leadership is to study recent international activity. President George Bush is known for his ability to maintain a dialogue and develop concerns among different factions in political and state decision making. He is also known to prefer dialogue to intervention as a problem-solving approach. These characteristics form part of his internal environment. When one of the republics of the Soviet Union declared its independence and was blockaded of crucial supplies as a result, Bush maintained a diplomatic dialogue with both the Soviet Union and the newly independent state of Lithuania. In a similar situation, John Kennedy, with a different internal environment, began an airlift of emergency supplies into Berlin when it suffered a similar blockade.

Paradoxically, George Bush's preference for dialogue was balanced in a different perspective when he considered and implemented a military invasion of Panama in 1989. The same leader, with the same internal values and preferred styles, acts very differently by balancing both internal and external forces.

Six Responsibilities of Effective Leadership

The remainder of this chapter will describe the roles of a leader in greater detail and explain how each role impacts manager effectiveness.

The Leader as Visionary

Managing the staff found in most health care departments presents challenges that are not unique to health care but

that are magnified by the high percentage of autonomous professionals typically found there. Effective management of professionals requires a manager to allow his staff the freedom to
establish their own work plans on a daily basis and to select, or at
least influence the selection of, the general approach to accomplishing their individual and team goals. By empowering staff to
accomplish goals in this manner, the manager-leader ensures
individual and group commitment to success.

Empowerment of a group of people to perform begins
with a common vision of the goal that the group must achieve.
Effective leaders develop a vision of success and communicate
this vision clearly to their followers. Although this vision may
require many small, individual contributions over a long period
of time to become reality, the leader must communicate her
vision in terms tangible and physically concrete.

Perhaps the most striking example in recent American
history of the power of shared vision to drive a team of followers
is that given by President Kennedy to the American people.
Kennedy's election in 1960 came shortly after several early tri-
umphs in space by the Soviet Union. While Kennedy's concerns
may have been partly related to nationalistic pride, they also ran
deeper in pragmatic concern about American security if there
were Soviet superiority in aerospace technology.

But this was not what Kennedy told the American people.
Nor did he share the potential for failure or the labor cost to
recapture technological superiority. What he said, as simply and
as forcefully as possible, was that the United States would place a
man on the moon within the decade.

Kennedy's vision was clear, and it was tangible enough to
survive the death of the visionary himself. The vision was one
easily conjured in the mind's eye, and powerful enough to drive
the entire nation to persevere through technological and personal tragedy resulting from many test failures and the deaths of
astronauts. Driven by that vision, the United States placed two
men on the moon in 1969. In health care there are many similar,
if quieter examples of the power of vision. In fact, many of the
nation's most enduring provider organizations, including Johns
Hopkins University Medical Center and the Baptist Health Sys-

tem, were begun by a small number of people who were able to share their vision with others.

The power of personal vision to drive individual efforts as well as group efforts has many examples in health care. It was a vision of curing polio that drove Jonas Salk for years to accomplish his goal and create the vaccine that now bears his name. It is personal vision, perhaps more than intellectual gift, that enables a college graduate to persevere through at least six years of grueling training to become a licensed physician in a particular field of practice.

But how does a manager develop a vision, and how can he effectively communicate that vision to his staff so that it can serve as a beacon to guide their work efforts? While the skill is easily learned, it requires great practice to master. The vision a manager creates for his department is built from a synthesis of many factors. Among the forces that mold a leader's vision is an understanding of the mission of the entire organization and the expectations of senior management for the department. The manager's vision must be consistent with this mission and the long-term expectations of institutional leaders. It would be pointless for a department manager to hold a vision of being a preeminent center for research if he were managing in a community hospital whose mission was to provide high-quality, low-cost care to the local population. There would be little support for the vision, and acting on it would create conflicts between the department and the provider when decisions were made regarding resource allocation and staffing issues. Another element shaping a leader's vision is an understanding of the direction of and developments in the manager's field of expertise. The manager who brings the possibilities of the larger world of her profession into her vision provides the challenge of accomplishment on a larger scale than what clinicians experience on a daily basis in most organizations. A fundamental principle of improving both education and human performance is that people will perform to whatever level of expectation is placed on them. Expect mediocrity and it will occur. Expect greatness and people will accomplish great things. By examining the larger world of her profession, and searching for greatness and the possibilities to be accomplished, the manager-leader brings these possibilities to her followers. And a third factor in a leader's vision involves the needs of the community served by the manager. What things can the manager strive for that will make the greatest impact upon those needs?

One of the better examples of how these forces influence a leader's vision is the story of the Jarvik heart. Robert Jarvik is a surgeon who worked for years trying to heal diseased hearts. Often, as is the case with chronic cardiopulmonary disease, his patients' hearts are simply too worn to continue, and donors are not readily available. Jarvik saw the need of his patients for a replacement for their worn hearts, and he saw the possibility of creating a completely artificial pump in the larger world of science. And when his vision to create this pump grew beyond the mission of his hospital, he found an organization whose mission was broad enough to contain his work. The message here is not to advocate leaving an organization when there is conflict but to demonstrate that the mission of an organization can influence the ideal vision for a leader who is part of that community.

One effective strategy for building a vision of success in a department requires the manager to close her eyes and create a mental image of the department at some point in the future. As the manager creates this vision, she should focus on visualizing the department after it has experienced its greatest success. The manager should focus on:

> Who is doing what in the department?
> > What types of people are on staff?
> > Are staff working as parts of teams that include other
> > > disciplines?
> > How is the manager spending her time?
> What services are being provided?
> > What client or patient needs have been met?
> > Which services are new and which are old?
> How are those services being delivered?
> > Are they centralized or decentralized?

As the manager creates this vision, she should focus upon creating in her mind as much detail as possible, including sounds. What do management peers and physicians say about the department? What do staff members say about working in the department?

This is the department that the manager will create. But to do this, she must have support and the focused effort of her staff and supervisors. Creating this vision has several practical applications, in addition to providing a mental image of success for the manager. By speaking to peers and superiors in terms of this vision, the manager can sensitize them to the potential for success and create in their minds an image of what that success looks like. Kennedy created an image of a man on the moon and all its associated glory in the minds of Congress, and it supported him. The health care leader, on a smaller scale, strengthens support for her vision by creating that vision in the minds of others.

Many effective leaders also use visualization to create a focus for staff energy. Some actually conduct visualization exercises with their staff to empower them with a vision of personal and group success. Why do this? After all, it is not what one might call "run-of-the-mill" management practice, and it certainly was not taught in "Departmental Administration 101." But this chapter is not about management. It is about leadership. Strong leaders have clear visions, and they communicate that vision to everyone they come in contact with. By inspiring others with a vision, a leader provides the direction for individual work and provides a common reason for striving. He also motivates peak performance if he can help others to see the big picture of departmental success as the goal of their daily detailed work.

Build and Maintain Trust

The word *trust* conjures images of security, predictability, and good will. We tend to think of trust in "degrees of existence." That is, if there is a high degree of trust, there is a high degree of cooperation, and effective work results from this. However, trust is a somewhat more complex issue for a leader. In reality, it is a function of consistency between statements and actions. It does not imply that there will be support and cooperative effort if there is a high degree of trust.

Therefore, a leader must consider trust a three-dimensional entity. The first dimension is the existence of trust. Generally, one can observe that trust does not exist when a leader's actions cannot be predicted based upon what she says. That is, simply because a leader says something will happen, his staff has no way of predicting whether, in fact, that will happen. The second dimension of trust is the nature of trust, which can be either constructive or destructive. If a manager is well known for not following through on promises, or for never acting on statements, his staff will clearly trust that when the manager says something, nothing will occur. To provide a simple example, if a nursing supervisor tells her staff that she will resolve a problem with the scheduling of routine X rays for patients when meals are delivered to patient rooms, and the problem continues, her staff will come to trust that when she says this, nothing will happen. There is trust, but not constructive trust.

A leader will depend heavily upon trust to encourage others to take risks and to pull together during difficult times. Constructive trust between individuals and groups, however, is a habitual response, developed after many small, seemingly unimportant experiences. If the aggregate of these experiences is positive, the trust between groups and a leader will be constructive. This does not mean that every statement of intent issued by a leader will come to pass. But when a leader says that he will do something, he is obligated to two actions: (1) attempting to complete the process he promised and (2) reporting to his staff in a timely manner the outcome of that attempt.

These two obligations, follow-through and communication, are essential elements for a leader who would build and maintain a high level of constructive trust. Both subjects are discussed in Chapter Three. Here, though, it is important to emphasize the imperative of consistency of both follow-through and communication in building trust. Because trust is a habitual response, and it can either be constructive or counterproductive, it is essential that the manager-leader develop as a habit the practice of immediate follow-through on statements with actions and that the results of those actions be communicated promptly to staff or others involved. This habit can be developed regardless of the style of one's leadership, and it will help ensure that a constructive trust exists.

Collaboration and Delegation as Trust-Building Practices. Beyond building a consistent pattern of action and communication, a manager-leader can develop other practices to build trust in her leadership. Two of the most effective methods are frequent collaboration with staff, peers, and superiors and effective use of delegation to accomplish goals.

Many traditional models of management accept and even promote intergroup collaboration as an effective way to create innovation and to solve problems affecting both groups. In many environments, this collaboration has been limited to the levels of management and at peer levels only. This is particularly true in industrial and corporate sectors of American business. In recent years, many management thinkers and, indeed, many practitioners have expanded the notion of collaboration as a problem-solving tool to include collaboration with managers and technical workers, both within a unit or department and between different departments. This collaboration has taken many forms, from expanding the use of democratic principles in planning, to the culturally popular self-managed work groups and the "skunk-works" philosophy written about extensively by Tom Peters in the *Wall Street Journal* and the *Baltimore Sun*.

Despite the positive results achieved by expanded use of the collaborative process, recent studies indicate that as many as 64 percent of American businesses still resist embracing this approach to managerial leadership (Takezawa and Whitehall, 1981). Perhaps not coincidentally, the competitive and creative standing of American business is still eroding. In a health care environment, collaboration is imperative for several reasons. The staff population of most departments is highly educated and has been professionally trained to diagnose and solve problems. A leadership style devoid of collaboration with this type of a staff is certain to have a negative effect upon the type of trust engendered. In addition to this consideration, the diverse and novel challenges facing departments require creative input and trusting support from all members of a group, leaders and followers alike.

The process of collaborating on planning and problem solving clearly identifies a greater number of solutions than a noncollaborative process does. In addition, while collaboration rarely produces a solution that is proposed and implemented without modification, each party in the process who is allowed to objectively criticize and offer constructive alternatives assumes ownership of and thus will support the final solution.

When is collaboration appropriate, and when is it not appropriate? Although there are no specific guidelines to make this determination, there are several models, ranging from conservative to extremely liberal, in reaching this decision. All of these models, however, have two things in common when employed successfully. First, they depend upon clear, consistent communication between the leader and other parties in the collaboration. This communication must be two way and collegial. Second, the collaboration must be allowed to serve its complete function. In other words, the leader cannot begin a collaborative process and then revert to rank-based decision making.

Intradepartmental collaboration models include the task force and the committee. Task forces are generally special-purpose groups formed to fulfill a specific function and then disbanded after that function is served. In this way they are similar in purpose to a project team, discussed in detail later in Chapter Six. An example of a task force might be one formed to identify and select the most effective strategy for expanding services to new consumers. The committee is generally an ongoing collaboration whose purpose is periodic assessment and recommendation regarding specific performance issues. For example, a committee might be established in a department for advising the leader about specific training needs and development needs as they see them emerging during the course of a year.

In addition to these traditional forms of collaboration, many institutions have experimented with establishing quality circles modeled after those implemented in manufacturing and other service industries. Quality circles are formalized structures that elicit the input of all employees to improve total quality of work (Mohr and Mohr, 1983). Experience with this formal structure is mixed in health care, however, with success apparently dependent upon the size of the organization and the commitment of senior administrators and physicians. This conclusion is based upon the experience of Japan, where implementation is generally simplified by the fact that in that culture, most senior administrative officers are also physicians.

I present delegation with collaboration as an essential strategy for building trust between the leader and his staff because delegation is the primary vehicle through which the leader shares his authority and associated responsibility. It is also one of the most challenging skills for a manager to master. A study conducted at the University of Michigan found that delegation was the most difficult aspect of leadership for 78 percent of a group of 2,500 people studied (Taylor, 1984).

Why is delegation such a persistent challenge? There are two essential issues for managers to confront in order to delegate effectively: (1) the leader's responsibility in delegation and (2) what should and should not be delegated.

The Leader's Responsibility in Delegation. Perhaps the most common error made in delegation is a leader's perception that his role is to carefully monitor and control delegated responsibilities. This is certainly an understandable confusion of responsibility. The health care manager is acutely aware of the ultimate accountability she has for decisions made and actions carried out within her department. Because of this sense of responsibility, there is often concern that "I need to have my hand in this, in order to make sure that everything proceeds well." The effect of this attitude toward delegation, however, is to send a message to subordinates that "I trust you, but I really don't quite trust you." This message, communicated to staff, creates a fear of failure and a lack of independent action.

One excellent example of this is the assistant administrator of a 450-bed hospital who also retained the title of chief operating officer for special services. He complained that he was no more than a glorified clerk and a "gofer" for the hospital administrator. When asked why he felt this way, he said that he apparently had profit-and-loss responsibilities for hundreds of thousands of dollars, but he could not hire a janitor without clearing it with the administrator. A review of some of his decisions revealed he had authority to make purchasing and patient care decisions. However, he was often overruled in important and relatively insignificant matters. He had been vetoed on purchasing a photocopier for secretarial staff, about changing staff assignments, and on buying new therapy equipment for the various services.

In this case, the administrator did not understand his essential role as a leader in effective delegation, and as a result, the assistant administrator felt untrusted and unimportant. The administrator's role should be one of communication and follow-up, not one of control. To be effective, delegation must be clearly communicated according to the following criteria. After determining what is to be delegated and to whom, the leader must communicate the following and confirm common understanding:

- What is expected to be produced (the final output)
- Any interim products (weekly status reports, for example)
- Follow-up schedules
- Scope of authority conveyed with the delegated task

Perhaps the most challenging of these four items is the last, scope of authority. In the example of the assistant administrator, the leader's lack of trust resulted in the assistant administrator having authority and then having that authority temporarily rescinded at the discretion of the leader, only to be returned later. This yo-yo phenomenon is a common threat to effective leadership. Once authority is delegated, it should remain with the person who is responsible for a task. The role of the leader after delegating a responsibility is not to control subsequent task completion, but to use follow-up communications as an opportunity to coach the now-responsible subordinate, providing advice based on the leader's greater experience with organizational process and technical completion of the responsibility. In this way, trust is built, the employee grows professionally, and the task is completed.

What to Delegate. In determining what responsibilities are best delegated, a manager might consider all of the things that must be done to manage a department, and group them in one of four categories. Relative to the manager's most personal responsibilities and his individual strengths and weaknesses, he should determine whether any given task or responsibility is:

   I.   Urgent and important
  II.   Not urgent but important
 III.   Urgent but not important
  IV.   Not urgent and not important

Activities that fall into category I are most important for the leader to manage personally. Tasks and activities that fall into category II are the most suitable for delegation to or collaboration with subordinates, peers, and superiors. Those in category III are most effectively delegated. Those in category IV can be delayed or delegated. This process, known as quadrant analysis, has the additional benefit of enabling the leader to quickly focus his attention on those matters that are most important for personal management, while providing direction about how to simultaneously accomplish other tasks. An example of how quadrant analysis might work for a manager in a health care setting is shown in Figure 2.2. This figure lists various tasks according to the manager's personal job priorities and where his individual talents are most needed.

How effectively do you delegate? Try the following questionnaire (Exhibit 2.1) to evaluate your skill as a delegator. Respond yes or no to its questions. An interpretation of your response follows the questionnaire.

Figure 2.2. Typical Quadrant Analysis—Department Manager.

I. Urgent–Important	II. Not Urgent–Important
• Explain budget variance to Chief Operating Officer this afternoon. • Respond to memo on Joint Commission on the Accreditation of Healthcare Organizations.	• Complete staff development plan. • Revise procedure manual.
III. Urgent–Not Important	IV. Not Urgent–Not Important
• Call family of Mrs. Doe: patient who complains that she is allergic to oxygen in nasal cannula.	• Lunch with neighbor at golf club.

Serve as a Political Conduit

Although trust and effective communication are essential to the leader's role as a political representative for his department and for the organization as a whole, they are not in themselves adequate preparation for this important responsibility. As a political agent for his department, the manager is responsible for monitoring events and developments in the organization that will affect specific plans or the entire department.

These factors include familiarity with cultural norms and taboos in the organization, awareness and intelligent use of the formal and informal power structure in the provider, and effective monitoring of changes in these areas. As political conduit, the manager ensures that key initiatives of the department receive political and resource support and that important department interests become important organizational interests.

Serve as Ethical Standard-Bearer for the Department

As mentioned earlier, effective leaders set standards of ethical conduct for their staff. Most health care managers readily

Exhibit 2.1. Delegation Effectiveness Questionnaire.

	Yes	No
1. Do I work long office hours? Do I take work home on a regular basis?	___	___
2. Do I work longer than my staff or fellow workers?	___	___
3. Do I spend time doing things for other people that they could do themselves?	___	___
4. In an emergency, is there a subordinate or colleague who could relieve me?	___	___
5. Do any of my colleagues, subordinates, or my boss know my work well enough to take over if I had to leave it?	___	___
6. Do I lack the time to plan my tasks and activities?	___	___
7. When I return from a business trip, is my desk piled high?	___	___
8. Do I still deal with activities or problems that were my responsibility before I got promoted?	___	___
9. Do I often have to postpone an important task to deal with others?	___	___
10. Am I constantly in a hurry in order to meet deadlines?	___	___
11. Do I spend time with routine work that could be done by someone else?	___	___
12. Do I dictate most of the correspondence, memos, and reports that I have to sign?	___	___
13. Do staff or peers often approach me with questions concerning meetings, projects, or tasks?	___	___
14. Do I lack time for social or company functions?	___	___
15. Do I want to be involved in and informed about everything?	___	___
16. Do I have a hard time following my priority list?	___	___

Interpreting your delegation effectiveness:
0–3 Yes Responses: Extremely effective delegator.
4–7 Yes Responses: Not bad, but could use some work.
8 + Yes Responses: This is an excellent opportunity to improve your personal effectiveness.

Source: Adapted from Seiwert (1989).

accept and understand the need for high standards of ethical conduct within their departments. The requirement for departmental ethics in action is broader than traditional standards that are incumbent on any clinical profession. Clinicians have been inculcated in their professional training and development with an understanding of personal ethics in care giving. The responsibility of a leader in maintaining standards for this behavior is generally not demanding because most professional clinicians have adopted and internalized an understanding of clinical ethics. This does not mean that the leader has no responsibility in maintaining clinical ethics at a high level in the department; the responsibility may require reinforcement of behavior that can be easily observed in many staff actions.

More challenging and more risky for the leader is to set a standard for managerial ethics within the department and in interdepartmental activities. Managerial ethics are in a state of flux for many providers. For example, it was once (and, arguably, still is) considered unethical to refuse care to any patient, regardless of ability to pay. This attitude is now being questioned. Many physicians and managers alike recognize the tragedy of refusing care. They also understand that to provide care to all who need it but who cannot pay can quickly undermine the responsibility to maintain fiscal viability for the community. The process of serving as an ethical standard bearer requires a leader to wrestle with the conflict created by these opposing understandings of what is the "right thing" to do. This example is a particularly difficult one for allied health managers, whose personal values direct them to act to provide care. This example is also used for its difficulty and to provide an illustration of the challenge facing leaders in health care at all levels. That challenge is to examine personal values and the ramifications of those values for determining the "right position" to take and the actions to implement in department policy and procedure.

Make Decisions

The leader's role as decision maker is one that requires balancing preferred style and situational effectiveness. To understand this more completely, you must understand the types of decision making that can occur on a daily basis. Lawrence Miller (1984) describes three types of decisions that are commonly made. First is the command decision. This type of decision is made autonomously, with little or no input from others in an organization. Examples of command decisions are those a nurse might make in the emergency room when faced with a severely bleeding patient and in the absence of a physician, who is preoccupied with an emergency in another care bay. Command decisions are generally effective over a short term and may not even be observed as "decisions" by managers or by those around them. The advantage of the command decision is its expediency at resolving issues quickly. One significant disadvantage of the command decision is that it may lead to a *functional* solution, but that solution is not always *optimal*.

The second type of decision making witnessed on a daily basis in most organizations is consultative decision making. Consultative decisions are made when a manager seeks input from peers and staff prior to making an independent decision. The manager who makes consultative decisions uses these sources of input to help evaluate alternatives and to provide information for decision making. There are several advantages to consultative decision making. The process is very effective when a manager must determine the impact of a decision on other areas of the organization. Consultative decisions are very helpful when "selling" ideas to other managers and physicians. One drawback to consultative decision making is if the process of consultation is misinterpreted as asking for permission to proceed. Compared to command decisions, consultative decisions require time and a knowledge of where in the organization opinions must be sought.

The third and potentially the slowest process of decision making is consensus decision making. Many American managers, particularly those in the health care field, find consensus decision making tiresome and risky. In consensus decision making, a leader turns responsibility for a decision over to a group, whose members must reach consensus about an issue. This process can be tiresome because it requires much more give-and-take between group members who must meet and closely collaborate, often over an extended period of time. The process can be risky because the manager relinquishes responsibility for the decision to the group, but is still left with accountability for the quality of that decision. On the other hand, consensus decision making is a powerful tool for reaching strategic decisions that will have a long-term impact on a department or on the provider organization.

Judge

The leader's responsibility to sit in judgment of a department or organization is one that carries with it both departmental and legal implications. Because of this and the fact that the leader who is a judge will then be asked to serve as a team leader and facilitator in subsequent situations, managers must support themselves and their staffs with clear, ongoing communication and documentation. Although specific circumstances requiring judgment cannot always be predicted, some generalizations can be made that will enable a leader to prepare people in a department for what to expect in any given situation. The most common situations requiring judgment include staff performance appraisal, quality assurance, and department-effectiveness audits. These and other universal situations of judgment within an organization can be facilitated with clear documentation of expectations. Examples of these are thorough policy and procedure manuals; documenting expected performance of people, equipment, and the organization in quantifiable terms; and specifying a range of consequences for substandard and above-standard performance. In the case of judgment of people, other tools to facilitate the leader's effectiveness are specified in Chapters Three and Eight.

One universal caveat regarding the role of a leader as judge is this: Responsibility cannot under any circumstances be passed to another individual, either within the department or outside of the department. Although the temptation to allow leadership responsibility to pass occasionally to another might be great, to give in to this temptation erodes the manager's credibility as a leader to both staff and peers. This does not mean that the manager cannot consider input provided by physicians, administrators, and others in an organization when judging events and individuals. It does mean, however, that the manager must clearly be seen as the individual who assesses all situations requiring judgment, and not merely as an agent of others in the organization.

Summary

No single approach to leadership is effective in every organization or in every situation. But the responsibility for leadership in a department clearly belongs with the manager. As leader, the manager must meet six responsibilities:

1. Be the source of a vision
2. Establish and maintain trust
3. Serve as political conduit
4. Serve as ethical standard-bearer for the department
5. Make decisions
6. Judge

These functions require the manager to use a variety of skills in every interaction, both within the department and with others elsewhere in the organization. This chapter has presented several of these leadership skills, including visualization, prioritization, collaboration, and delegation. The next chapter explores the leader's most frequently used skill — communication.

3

Communicating Effectively: *Up, Down, and Across the Organization*

by Joseph G. Sorbello*

No single aspect of the manager's job can contribute to career success as much as being an effective communicator. Managers operate in a social environment and are judged by their ability to deal with people: superiors, fellow managers, employees, and persons outside their management environment. It is often difficult to find a good, practical resource to complement your previous training and experience in communicating with others. This chapter is designed to be a resource of materials, information, and guidelines to help health care managers become more effective communicators.

The focus of this chapter is on the how-tos of everyday communication. They include:

- Formulating effective written and oral messages to three audiences: employees, peers, and upper management
- Recognizing and managing barriers to communication
- Measuring your own communication effectiveness

*Joseph G. Sorbello is assistant professor, Programs in Respiratory Care and Cardiorespiratory Sciences, College of Health Related Professions, State University of New York Health Science Center at Syracuse.

- Applying a knowledge of personality profiles described in Chapter Two to strengthen communication
- Strengthening your listening skills
- Using to your advantage existing institutional channels of communication, including the grapevine and the rumor mill

Communication can be defined as the active process of sharing meanings. It is a process that requires work both by the sender and the receiver. This involves our total behavior, from actually uttering words to making subtle physical gestures that enhance what we have to say. How we achieve shared meanings is often difficult to analyze.

Written Communication: Employees, Peers, and Upper Management

In any form of communication, particularly the written form, you must carefully consider with whom you are communicating. In most instances, the format and style with which you communicate with an employee will differ greatly from the way you communicate with a superior. Figure 3.1 shows a management communication model demonstrating the nature of managerial communication, the role of the manager, and the role of the person to whom the manager is communicating. Where communication is concerned, be sure to remember the managerial criteria of effectiveness, efficiency, and quality. Your choices of both message and channel will greatly influence what is actually communicated to your audience.

Written communication does not provide the instant feedback that oral communication provides. Therefore, written communication must, by nature, be more carefully designed to ensure that the message is clearly understood. Also, written messages can be retained as references or legal records. Remember that once something is in writing, it is very difficult, if not impossible, to retract. Managers should be extra cautious in determining the message and channel options when communicating through the written word.

Figure 3.1. A Model for Managerial Communication.

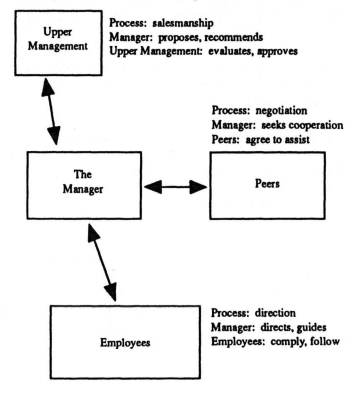

Try these simple guidelines when communicating in writing with employees:

- Be decisive in your communication. Project a positive and authoritative (not cocky) attitude. Your writing should direct the employee and let him or her know that you are in control of the situation. Besides eliminating nearly all doubt as to the purpose of the communication, this will tend also to express to your employees your confidence in your abilities as a manager.
- As one of the first written communications to employees, publish and make available to all employees a document that states clearly your expectations of him or her on a daily

basis. This may simply be a standard evaluation form, or it may involve many statements and forms, depending on the institution or setting.

- Whenever an employee is given a major project to do, the details should be written down and agreed upon, especially the deadlines. The employee and manager should each have a copy of this agreement.

Follow these guidelines when writing to peers:

- Remember that some peers may be your friends and some may be competing with you for real or imagined future positions. The style or tone of your communication rather than the actual content may become the message of your communication. To this end, all peer-to-peer communication should reflect a spirit of cooperation and of collegiality.
- Note that you are not trying to direct someone's activity but rather create a cooperative atmosphere. It is important not to appear dominant or aggressive when communicating with peers, particularly since much written communication to peers will be to ask for input and support.

When writing to upper management, keep these points in mind:

- Always remember to equate communication with upper management with salesmanship.
- You should be recommending actions, not asking your boss to manage your area.
- Clearly state the problem or situation, establish alternatives, and always propose a final recommendation or next step. Be succinct and precise.
- Use written communication as a tool to prepare your superior. For example, if you anticipate a call for some of your personnel to "float" to another floor or area of the hospital because of a critical shortage, you could supply a potential list of these people and what impact such transfers would have on your department or unit. Then, when your super-

visor is approached by his peer, he will be ready with an answer. This will indicate a well-organized operation and reflect well on you and your supervisor.

As examples of written communication, let us examine three memoranda by Emily Foley, a middle-level manager. The general subject is the same for all three examples: the completion of a proposal for outpatient services. The process of communication in these memos is the one outlined in Figure 3.1. Each of these memos is effective, but you will notice a different tone of communication with each.

Memo to Employee

To: Victor Fong
From: Emily Foley
As you know from my most recent staff meeting, it is a priority for you to complete the Outside Services Proposal on schedule. From our last status review, I'm not convinced that this is possible. I strongly encourage you to take Keith or Donna from their current time study project and put them on this task for the next two weeks. I am willing to accept a late completion of the time study but not for the Outside Services Proposal.

Memo to Peer

To: Alma Rodriguez
From: Emily Foley
As you know from yesterday's lunch discussion, I am in the middle of trying to complete the Outside Services Proposal. We are behind schedule, and I need two additional nurses for half time to complete the proposal in two weeks. I recall you mentioning that you are in a slack period right now and, therefore, I'm wondering if I could enlist your support for the next two weeks and borrow Keith and

Donna half time. After the Outside Services Proposal is complete, I will be done with the computers I am currently using. Based on my discussion, I know that your work on the Medicaid project is limited by your ability to produce the numbers needed for your justifications. Therefore, early completion of the Outside Services Proposal will ensure that the resources needed for your Medicaid project are available. I truly appreciate your help in this matter.

Memo to Upper Management

To: Brian Kirk
From: Emily Foley

I have recently reviewed the work for the Outside Services Proposal. To complete the proposal on schedule, two additional steps need to be taken: adding manpower and getting computer time priority. I have taken action to reassign people within my groups to help in this effort. The main problem right now is computer time priority. I have tried Frank Kieffer, the new computer services manager, to get the needed priority, but due to prior demands upon the computer, he cannot support this effort for the next three weeks. I believe that the most effective way to manage this roadblock would be to get Jim Metzberg to place this project as a priority for computer time. While I will be happy to do this, I believe that you would be more effective at this, since both of you are vice presidents.

All three memos communicate the same basic message, but the tone and style differ because of the differences in communication level and the desired outcome for each communication.

Oral Communication:
Employees, Peers, and Upper Management

In contrast to written communication, oral communication is more personal and provides instant feedback, through oral responses and body language. It is true that actions often speak louder than words, and body language can convey much more than what you say. For example, a person who insists that he is not angry is not always convincing, especially when pounding the table or delivering his message with a glare. Often it is difficult for people to know what kind of body message they are sending along with the spoken word. Some general guidelines follow for effective oral communication with employees, peers, and superiors. Although the following suggestions are geared toward dealings with employees, you may want to keep them in mind when communicating with peers, upper management, and others outside of the work environment.

- Set up a formal plan with communications held at regular intervals. People want to know what is happening, and even more important, they need to make themselves heard. A regular schedule of communication with staff fulfills these needs and provides you with important operational status information.
- Whenever possible, use reason, logic, and persuasion rather than direction to influence employees.
- In addition to formally scheduled communication sessions, consider establishing an open-door policy. Create an atmosphere so that employees are not afraid to come to see you. However, make sure they know that there will be times when you will be unavailable for even short meetings.
- Ask the employee for his or her views, including suggestions for improving the situation. Then, offer any suggestions you might have. Next, agree upon actions to be taken and schedule more meetings if you think review is required.
- Do not solve problems that employees should be solving themselves. Offer suggestions on how they might resolve the problems, but do not commit time to helping them solve

their dilemma. Instead of saying, "Let me think about that and get back to you," try saying, "I'll consider your problem, but you must continue working on this in the meanwhile. In fact, you should also develop some alternatives and get back to me by the fifteenth, so we can discuss what you've come up with." This makes it absolutely clear that the responsibility for completion is where it should be.

In communicating orally with peers, remember these points:

- Do not put them in an employee position. A collegial or negotiating posture rather than a directive or counseling approach is needed.
- Consider how your actions and decisions affect the operation of other departments. Make decisions that will benefit rather than hinder them.
- Recognize that other managers have goals and commitments, and realize they have problems just as you do. Treat them as partners rather than opponents. Offer to help whenever you have an opportunity. This, in turn, puts you in a good position for reciprocal cooperation, should you need it.

Consider these guidelines when talking to upper management:

- Because the time with your superior will probably be limited, always be prepared ahead of time. First, gather all the information that is relevant to the discussion. Briefly outline what you want to present, while remembering your manager's style and the position he or she has taken on previous issues.
- During your meeting, start by stating specifically what you want to discuss and the reasons for your concern. Mention relevant actions or conditions, and explain why you are bringing them to his attention.

- Follow up by presenting the courses of action you have considered and your evaluation of each of them. Next, ask your manager for any comments he or she might have, then agree upon a plan.
- When you return to your office, summarize your meeting by writing down all the important points covered; store this for future reference. This suggestion is meant for *all* oral communication, particularly with upper management.

Assessing the Effectiveness of Communication

There are many useful systems for evaluating the quality of ongoing communications between a manager and his staff and between the manager and others in the organization. The questionnaire in Exhibit 3.1 is a simple and effective way to determine the general quality of communication. It can be used to assess communication between both staff and superiors in an organization.

To evaluate communication, follow this two-step process:

1. Have all managers and supervisors in a department complete the questionnaire from the perspective of staff. That is, they should answer all questions as they think the staff would answer them. Then compile the results by item.
2. Have the staff complete the same questionnaire anonymously, compile the results, and then compare the differences and similarities between the groups.

In addition to the scoring guidelines for interpretation of individual scores, which follow, any significant disparity between the responses of the two groups indicates a need to focus on the quality of communication between staff and management in a department.

Count up the number of Y's circled. If you have ten, your communication with your manager is just about perfect. Nine or eight indicates good communication, seven or six is above average, and five or less needs improvement.

Exhibit 3.1. A Communication Tool: Your Own Barometer.

Here's a quick way to measure the quality of your communication with your manager. Read the following questions, and circle either Y (for Yes) or N (for No).

Y   N   1. I can ask for help without feeling embarrassed.

Y   N   2. My manager recognizes the good things I do.

Y   N   3. I understand what my manager expects of me.

Y   N   4. My manager coaches me toward improvement when I need it. .

Y   N   5. I am aware of the reasons for the major decisions my manager has made this year.

Y   N   6. My manager understands my personal goals.

Y   N   7. I know at least two specific things I can do to get a better rating at my next performance review.

Y   N   8. My manager lets me know when I miss the mark, but without putting me down.

Y   N   9. I feel free to disagree with my manager when we talk.

Y   N   10. My manager is aware of the basic problems I have to cope with in doing my job.

Source: Reproduced with adaptation from *Practical Supervision* by permission of the publisher, Professional Training Associates, Inc.

Understanding Personality Types to Improve Communication

Many organizations, including hospitals and other health care facilities, have used the Myers-Briggs Type Indicator (MBTI) to profile personality types. These types will be presented as a vehicle for improving the effectiveness of teams in Chapter Six, but understanding the individual differences among peers, staff, and superiors can strengthen communications as well. What follows is a discussion of how managers can apply an understanding of personality types in day-to-day communication. Note, however, that before applying this understanding, one must acquire the understanding. To this end, managers are encouraged to employ either the MBTI or similar profiling systems to enhance department effectiveness. The guidelines and implications that follow complement the process of profiling and do not replace profiling.

The Myers-Briggs Type Indication system measures personality types across four continua:

1. *Extroversion/Introversion* profiles how a person interacts with the environment to become "energized." The premise is simple—certain types of people have a preference for interacting with the external environment and find that interaction refreshing and energizing. Others prefer contemplative activities, solitary thought, and consideration. This does not mean that an introvert by preference cannot or does not enjoy interacting with others; it means that given a choice of any activity to engage in, he or she will opt for an introverted type of activity.

2. *Sensing/Intuiting* is a gauge of how a person gathers meaningful information. A person with a preference for sensing likes to gather information that is immediate and empirical and that can be validated with the five senses. A person with an intuitive preference relies more on the interpreted meaning of information gathered from the world. Intuitive people will assimilate information, but to them the importance of that information is in its meaning or relationship to other information. To communicate effectively with a "sensor," simply present bare-bones, logical empirical evidence. To communicate effectively with an "intuitor," translate data into a statement of implications.

3. *Thinking/Feeling* evaluates what influences a person's decision-making process. A thinker abstracts personal considerations and the personal implications for others in making a decision. The thinker values logic and fact when making decisions. The person with a feeling preference brings into his process of evaluation the personal implications for himself and others of information and situational developments on a day-to-day basis. As with the other continua, people with one preferred style can function in the other mode, but their preferred style will influence their

actions and how to most effectively communicate with them.

4. *Judging/Perceiving* measures how people interact in making decisions as well as how they prefer to resolve problems, among other things. A person with a preferred style of judging wants to reach final consensus or problem resolution and be done with an issue. The judging preference leads to reaching decisions rapidly and bringing issues to a close. The perceiving preference in people leads to a more adaptive style of problem resolution and greater consideration of multiple contingencies and compromise.

Within these continua are sixteen discretely defined type combinations (see Figure 6.2 in Chapter Six). This model for typing personality is perhaps the most thoroughly validated. Its implications are significant for team selection, management of interpersonal conflict, and communication. This section will focus on how a manager can use a knowledge of MBTI types to more effectively communicate on the job.

Communication involves interpretation. We have a tremendous capacity to edit, rearrange, omit, judge, and interpret the messages we receive. Interpretations are influenced by our preferences of extroversion or introversion. According to Carl Jung, we are all both introverted and extroverted. But in most of us, one aspect is preferred and controls more of our behavior: "When we consider the course of human life, we see how the fate of one individual is determined more by the objects of his interest [extrovert], while in another it is determined more by his own inner self, by the subject [introvert]. Since we all swerve rather more towards one side or the other, we naturally tend to understand everything in terms of our own type. . . . In respect of one's own personality one's judgment is as a rule extraordinarily clouded" (Jung, 1976, p. 3). Remember that while each element of personality type influences how we communicate, the most significant of these may be what determines our preferred way of interacting with the outside world: extroversion-introversion.

Extrovert Versus Introvert

Extroverts prefer people, activities, and the external environment. They are largely energized by stimuli from the external environment. Their attention flows outward to people, objects, and activities to maximize interaction. They perceive and judge from this perspective predominantly. Introverts prefer privacy and the inner world of ideas, beliefs, and ordered existence. Introverts are energized by internal stimuli of order and meaning; their attention flows inward. Introverts withdraw attention from the external world in order to balance and establish internal order. They perceive and judge primarily from this point of view.

Let us look at some basic preference differences between extroverts and introverts:

Extroverts	*Introverts*
Outside world	Inner world
People, action, things	Ideas, thoughts, meanings
Interaction	Reflection
Usually talkative and outgoing	Usually quiet and reserved
Sociable with many friends	Introspective with a few close
Refers to others as friends	friends — discriminates clearly between acquaintance and friend
Tends to like meeting new people	Tends to postpone meeting new people
Sociable	Territorial
External events	Internal reactions
Tends to expand rather than conserve — expansive	Tends to consolidate, defend and protect — avoids personal disclosure
Reacts to stress primarily by increasing activity	Reacts to stress primarily by decreasing activity

Energized by activity   Energized by depth and
                                   intimacy

In looking at the differences in preference, several things stand
out. The extrovert deals with space, time, territory, and interaction differently from the introvert. Let us examine some
extrovert-introvert behaviors and strategies in order to explore
implications for effective communication.

Lee and Norma Barr have written an excellent text, *The
Leadership Equation* (1989) on the use of the MBTI, and I highly
recommend it for health care managers and leaders. In their
management workshops, they asked extroverts and introverts to
identify what they like about each other, what they dislike, and
what advice they would give each other for improving communication. These are some of the characteristics they value about
each other:

Extroverts	*Introverts*
Make quick decisions	Make well-thought-out decisions
Brainstorming capability	Have concentration depth
Gather information quickly	Gather information thoroughly
Straightforward	Responsible, in-depth opinions
Talk easily	Use discretion in talking
Stimulate communication	Focus on subject matter at hand and bring talk back to the topic
Do not mind interruptions	Longer attention span
Good in spontaneous response	Persuasive with sound logic
Able to switch gears easily	Tenacious, serious, focused
Good at group social interaction	Good at one-to-one interaction
Good at stimulating ideas	Good at developing ideas
Enthusiasm and energy level	Calmness and quiet

Instigate action   Keep confidences

In these workshops, as groups began to think about the differences between extroverts and introverts, the strengths of both
began to come out. Appreciation of differences is essential for
communication. A leader uses the strengths of each, knowing
just the right mix of styles to maximize productivity. The advice
offered by both groups provides fertile ground for developing
everyday management strategies.

Extroverts' Advice to Introverts for Communication

- Be assertive.
- Express your ideas.
- Show your emotion—let others see you as human.
- Be friendly, talk more.
- Be open-minded.
- Be more upbeat, show a more lively nature.
- Invite us to an activity once in a while. Do not make us do all
  the arrangements.
- Do not take things too seriously.
- Smile more. You are hard to approach.
- Be more playful. Do not worry about what others think.
- Give more information on where you are on an issue.
- Tell me if you like or dislike what I am saying.
- Do not judge me as frivolous just because I am extroverted.
- Be flexible.

Introverts' Advice to Extroverts for Communication

- Respect our privacy. Do not take up our space.
- Do not put us in the spotlight.
- Do not demand an immediate response. Give us the infor-
  mation and let us have time to digest it.
- Tone down. Do not overwhelm us with your bluster.
- Pay closer attention to what we are saying.
- Give us more facts and less small talk.
- Help us feel more comfortable by not judging us as inferior.
  Remember that not everyone acts the same.

- Do not betray something we told in confidence.
- Learn to listen. Be more understanding of other people's need to express themselves. Just because we will not fight you for center stage does not mean that we do not have something to say.
- Put your brain in gear before your mouth takes off.
- Be patient. It takes longer for us to express ourselves.
- Do not patronize us.
- Let us know which ideas you are really serious about and that you are genuinely committed to follow through.
- Do not judge us as dull just because we are quiet.
- Follow through when we agree to do something. You seem to be always looking for a better offer. It seems you will work with me if you cannot find someone more interesting.

Both groups can improve communication with each other by remembering a few points. Introverts need to keep in mind that extroverts prefer the social and active, and are mainly focused on the external environment. Introverts can also modify their behavior by giving feedback and showing interest, emotion, and involvement. They should try to respond more both verbally and nonverbally and suspend their annoyance with "nonpurposeful" talk. Value can come from interacting rather than the quality of ideas exchanged. While introverts should attempt to respond more quickly and spontaneously, they should also avoid talking too long at one time. Extroverts prefer short bursts rather than long monologues.

To improve communication with introverts, extroverts should remember that introverts prefer the private and serious, but they often have a very sophisticated sense of humor. Extroverts can adjust their behavior by respecting privacy and not asking personal questions that invade private psychological space. They should also try to give introverts time to think about ideas or decisions and ask for specific information—introverts may not give it, unless asked. In addition, extroverts should think before speaking, slow down, and pay close attention to what introverts are saying and doing; they tend to give subtle signals that extroverts often overlook.

Your natural preferences for introversion or extroversion may be strong. Effective communication will result from an understanding of the differences between the types and of the implications for effectively communicating with both.

Sensor Versus Intuitor

Our preference for sensory or intuitive information affects how we see the world. People with a strong sensory preference prefer to gauge the world through their five senses. They are most comfortable focusing on the present and interpreting anything new by what they have already experienced or can validate with physical sensation. Their counterparts, the intuitors, interpret information according to its meaning, possibility, and implication. Sensors focus on what someone *said*. Intuitors focus on what they *meant*. Let us look at their different characteristics:

Sensor	*Intuitor*
Practical	Idealistic
Concrete	Abstract
Realistic	Conceptual
Focused on today	Focused on tomorrow
Prefers factual interpretation	Prefers "possibility" interpretation
Tends to be physically competitive	Tends to be intellectually competitive
Produces steadily	Produces cyclically
Results oriented	Idea oriented
Dislikes change	Likes variety and challenge
Sensible	Imaginative
Prefers step-by-step specific routine	Prefers overall or holistic viewpoint
Dislikes ambiguity	Dislikes rigid situations

Dislikes long-range planning   Dislikes too much structure
Prefers concrete examples   Prefers symbols, concepts,
and facts   and meanings

Now consider the differences between the sensor and intuitor and how they process information. The way we manage information can increase or decrease our power to produce. Sensors prefer to test ideas, examine facts, and complete tasks. Intuitors would rather generate ideas, follow instincts, and make improvements. Sensors are cautious and linear and tend to have a preprogrammed viewpoint according to norms and experience. Intuitors are quick and intuitive and generally look for a fresh view. Neither way of perceiving is correct or incorrect. However, there are strengths and weaknesses of both that have implications for communication. Let us examine these for the sensor and intuitor:

Sensor

Strengths	*Weaknesses*
Likes observable facts	May overlook implications and meanings
Likes information explained step by step	May not see the guiding principle behind the information
Prefers the practical, realistic, and present	May reject new, innovative ideas and may not see future demands in time
Likes to get things done	May cut too many corners, push too hard, and do things too quickly
Commands others; orders others	May not discuss or ask enough questions or take the time to build group support

| Likes competition | May compete over unimportant issues, may perceive noncompetitive situations as win-lose situations |

Intuitor

Strengths	*Weaknesses*
Thinks quickly; reads between the lines	May skim information and miss essential variables and omit facts
Uses "big picture" thinking while synthesizing random data	May leave things dangling or be scattered and unfocused
Conceptualizes easily, sees possibilities, and recognizes patterns	May overrate possibilities and focus on secondary instead of primary issues
Is visionary and individualistic	May be impractical, too independent, and egocentric

Now that we know the basic characteristics, strengths, and weaknesses of the sensors and intuitors, let us examine some tested strategies for enabling both to understand the perspective of each other. This understanding will facilitate effective communication between them.

Strategies for the Sensor

1. Learn to get quiet and focus internally.
2. Practice deep breathing as a method of slowing down, relaxing, and looking internally.
3. Select an external sensory object, close your eyes, and let your intuitive mind play with the object. Do not control or judge; let the intuitive mind expand, flow, and invent ways of looking at the object.

4. Observe several people in a room. Consciously see the pattern in which they are standing. See the objects in the room as colors only, or in hues ranging from light to dark, or in terms of tall or short.
5. Unfocus attention to the details of a situation and see what it reminds you of. Let the mind produce some associations, some patterns.

Strategies for the Intuitor

1. Focus on the task at hand, establish a time limit, and stick to it.
2. Discipline yourself to concentrate on one thing at a time. Try focusing on several objects in a room one at a time. You will probably notice yourself quickly start to scan and cluster things together. Slow down and discipline yourself to really see each object. Notice consciously the shapes, colors, textures, configurations. Make yourself attend to detail.
3. Think about a person. Go deeper than the flood of impressions and feelings until you begin to see. Practice trying to recall specific details about that person.
4. Focus on some work you are doing. See it as it is, right at this moment. Stop yourself from racing ahead to how to change it or improve it. See it now.
5. See if you can turn off the internal noise, relax, breathe deeply, and go beyond mental activity to internal stillness.

Thinker Versus Feeler

We perceive through sensing-intuiting channels, and we make decisions about our perceptions through thinker-feeler channels. This way of judging affects how we prefer information to be presented. The thinker judges according to rationality of the information. A feeler judges according to the personal application of the information. The thinker values logical organization, and the feeler values personal rapport with the information. Thinkers and feelers are often in conflict with each other because each presents information as they would prefer to receive it. When the thinker presents a feeler with concrete, logically structured information but no specific treatment of the "big picture" implications, communication is less than effective. The reverse is also true for the feeler who presents information that is replete with interpretation and conclusion, but sparse in supportive logic. The following summary of the strengths and weaknesses of each type have specific implications for communication.

Feeler

Strengths	*Weaknesses*
Shares emotional sensitivity	May collect too much emotional data and become overloaded with feelings that distort accurate perception
Behaves demonstratively and expressively	May give away too much information, time, and energy
Sees the people perspective; interprets events as they affect people	May oversimplify and overpersonalize
Charms and persuades	May rely too much on charm and not enough on preparation
Can hook people's initial interest	May take too long getting to the main point; may be too imprecise to get the message across
Gives a descriptive account of a situation or event	May tell too many anecdotes and stories
Likes to communicate	May spend too much time talking

Thinker

Strengths	*Weaknesses*
Prefers the analytical, logical expression	May analyze instead of internalize while trying to avoid emotional expression

Values logic	May undervalue feelings in motivating people
Handles emergencies logically	May appear cold, insensitive
Explains thoroughly and probes deeply	May overexplain and ask too many questions
Prefers to keep remarks objective and impersonal	May try to suppress feelings; may appear insincere
Likes a formal approach	May be overly formal

Goals and Strategies for Thinkers and Feelers

In trying to balance the characteristics, strengths, and weaknesses of each, try establishing the following goals. Thinkers need to integrate feelings into their rationale without letting feelings dominate or control rationale. Feelers should integrate clear cause-and-effect thinking into their rationale. Both thinkers and feelers should try to master the following strategies:

- Attend to personal associations and feelings as part of the understanding of a situation or person; attend to principles, variables, and facts in the cause-effect relationships of the situation.
- Appreciate as well as evaluate.
- Avoid habitual skepticism or blind optimism by clearly assessing both positive and negative aspects of situations.
- Integrate objectivity and compassion.
- Express affection as well as criticism.
- Evaluate when exceptions to a rule are equally as valid as the rule.
- Personalize as well as analyze.

Judge Versus Perceiver

The way we control is affected by our judging or perceiving preference. A strong judging preference indicates a desire to decide, evaluate, plan, organize, and maximize use of time. Perceivers have a desire to adapt, respond, decide outcomes, and adjust as they go. Preference for judging or perceiving affects the communication channels. Judge preference tags the judgment channels of thinker or feeler as the dominant channel, while perceiver preference indicates that sensor or intuitor will be the dominant channel. Our development as workers, managers, or ultimately as leaders is affected by our natural preferences of communication, information processing, judging, and controlling. Here are the critical attributes of the judging type and the perceiving type that most influence their approach to communication:

Judge	*Perceiver*
Wants to finish	Wants to stay open to something new
Controls time	Controls own participation
Prefers advance notice	Enjoys spontaneity
Prefers decisiveness	Prefers to postpone decisions to see if they really need to be made
Wants only essential information for the plan	Wants ample information to explore more options
Decides and plans	Adapts and changes
Is goal oriented	Is process oriented
Can jump to conclusions too quickly just to reduce ambiguity and get closure	Can postpone decisions too long, get pulled in too many directions, and be too scattered to decide

Communication with people who prefer either type is best composed and provided by understanding what that person is likely to value and prefer. This does not mean that a person with a preference for judging should not be approached with a perceiving message of the alternatives and implications; it means that the message should present the problem, state the recommended action, and then follow that with additional information.

The four continua presented by the Myers-Briggs Type Inventory provide a powerful, yet easily understandable framework for proactively planning communication and diagnosing problems in communicating with various people in an organization. Such a system allows one to examine ineffective and effective communication and to compensate for differences in individual styles.

Listening as a Component of Communication

Every effective model of communication includes a sender and a receiver of a message. In day-to-day communication, the reception of messages is accomplished by listening. Effective listening often enables a manager to receive communication that may be unintentional but crucial to understanding what is being expressed.

There are four general types of listeners: the nonlistener, marginal listener, evaluative listener, and active listener. Each type requires a particular depth of concentration and sensitivity on the part of the listener. As one advances among these levels, the potential for understanding, trust, and effective communication increases. You can identify these four types by recognizing the characteristics of each: The nonlistener does not hear the person or try to listen. Although nervous mannerisms and blank stares may give her away, she fakes attention while thinking about unrelated matters. She is busy preparing what she wants to say and constantly interrupting the speaker. Perceived as a social bore and a know-it-all, the nonlistener must always have the last word.

The marginal listener hears sounds and words but may miss the meaning. He stays on the surface of a conversation and is easily distracted. The marginal listener prefers to evade difficult or technical discussions; when listening to these discussions, he listens only for the bottom-line facts rather than main ideas. Despite verbal and nonverbal cues that he is listening, he is not.

The evaluative listener hears the speaker but does not try to understand the speaker's intent. She tends to be a logical listener, more concerned with content than feelings, and remains emotionally detached from the conversation. Adept at repeating verbatim words just delivered, she ignores the message conveyed in the speaker's voice tone, body language, and facial expressions. The evaluative listener anticipates a person's words and is ready with a retort before that person is finished speaking. Because she forms opinions about the message before it is complete, she risks misunderstanding it.

The active listener attempts to see things from other people's point of view by placing himself in their position. He pays attention to the content of others' messages as well as to their intent and feeling. Instead of interrupting others, he constantly looks for verbal and visual cues indicating that they would like to say something. The active listener is aware of what is and is not said. He is also a skillful questioner, using questions to encourage others to extend the conversation and clarify their message. By probing areas that need to be developed further, he tries to get a total picture of what others (employees, peers, or superiors) are trying to communicate.

The active listener, clearly the ideal, exhibits three skills the other types of listeners lack: sensing, attending, and responding. *Sensing* is the ability to recognize and appreciate the silent messages from the speaker such as vocal intonation, body language, and facial expressions. *Attending* refers to verbal, vocal, and visual messages that the listener sends to the speaker indicating attentiveness, receptiveness, and acknowledgment of the speaker and message. *Responding* occurs when the active listener attempts to obtain feedback on the accuracy of his understanding, keep the speaker talking, gather more information, and make the speaker feel understood. The goal of a communicator should be to foster active listeners in your organization, including yourself. Encourage others to improve themselves; this will make the job of communication easier. The following list of ideas suggested by Nichols and Stevens (1986) is meant to help people, particularly managers, become better listeners. Of course, not all of these suggestions are applicable to every organization or situation. The most important thing, however, may be not what happens when a specific suggestion is followed but rather what happens when people become aware of the problem of listening and of what specific improvements in their listening skills they can demonstrate.

- Devote an executive seminar, or seminars, to a discussion of the roles and functions of listening as a management tool.
- Use filmed cases for management training programs. Cases present the problem as it would appear in reality, and viewers are forced to practice good listening habits to be sure of what is going on. This includes not only hearing the sound track but also watching the facial mannerisms, gestures, and motions of the actors.
- Bring in qualified speakers and ask them to discuss listening with special reference to how it might apply to management. Such speakers are available at universities where listening is taught as a part of communication training.
- Give a self-scored test in listening ability.
- In a training session, hold a conference on a selected problem and tape-record it. Afterward, play back the recording. Discuss it in terms of listening. Do the contributions of different participants reflect good listening? If the conference should go off the track, try to analyze the causes in terms of listening.
- If there is time after a regularly scheduled conference, hold a listening critique. Ask each member to evaluate the listening attention that he received while talking and to report his analyses of his own listening performance.

Networking

An effective manager is a master at building, maintaining, and nurturing a network of communication that not only will, in effect, enhance the manager's image as a good communicator but also will help to make the organization work more efficiently and effectively. Networking involves sharing information and services among people with a common interest. It is a system for sharing. The benefits of networking for a manager include:

- Sources of information: Information changes quickly in the health care world. Networking can connect you with current developments in technology and information.
- Sources of expertise: Some expertise is more readily available through the ideas and experience of other individuals.
- Sources of job/career opportunities: Information on job openings is often available internally long before it is published in journals, newspaper want ads, or sent to personnel recruiters. Most jobs are filled without ever going public.
- Sources of business opportunities: Leaders, managers, consultants, and other professionals use their networks to find leads about possible business opportunities and access to organizations.
- Sources of consultants and vendors: Professionals regularly use their networks to identify consultants, subcontractors, and vendors appropriate to their needs. Besides supplying names, networks can provide evaluations and recommendations.
- Sources of insight/advice to better solve problems: Network members are frequently used as sounding boards. Respected members of the network are asked for their opinions, experience, and perspectives in relation to a specific problem being faced.
- Sources of marketability data: Promotions, job changes, and political realities within organizations are common network gossip. They provide comparative data by which to assess your marketability beyond your current position.

Most managers probably have not consciously constructed an intricate and goal-directed communication network. However, most would probably agree that they already have a network in place without realizing it. If you lack a network or have not thought about strengthening your existing network, here are some suggestions that you might try to follow in a systematic way to get your network into shape (Hutchison, 1988).

Meet new people, exchange business cards, and get to know current colleagues better. Talk to people you already know, and ask questions. Make connections whenever you are able. Sometimes it is difficult to determine who will be able to help you with a specific problem or who will be an asset to continued networking. Be aware of the potential with every contact you make, both social and professional. In your conversations, remember to use active listening skills. Analyze what is being said for potential networking opportunities, even if at the moment you are unable to connect them with a resource or offer any assistance. Try to reach a level beneath the surface conversation where you may discover networking opportunities that less experienced ears may not detect. Are you familiar with similar projects or problems? What kind of information and expertise would have been helpful for you in a similar situation? If you were the person talking, what would you want or need?

As you gather information, file away what you hear. Either file it in your memory if you are skilled at that type of recall, or write it down in a file devoted to networking opportunities. This file may need to be subdivided as your network expands. Make connections between similar topics, problems, and opportunities. Periodically review your file. Look for opportunities to connect one individual with another. Check that you have not left commitments hanging uncompleted. And while you assess others' value, establish your value to your network. Everyone has something to offer to a network. If you are new to the field, you can always offer to do research or administrative tasks on a project and help someone else while you are expanding your own knowledge. Update your network on your areas of expertise, interest, and experience. Provide tips and leads that you think your network members can benefit from. Keep abreast of activity within the field. As you learn, keep applications to your network in mind.

At professional conferences and through notes and phone calls, keep in touch with the members of your network. When you know colleagues will be contacting mutual acquaintances, have them say hello for you. Even this keeps your name and activities visible within your network. Read professional literature and newsletters dealing with management science and the health care industry; listen to your conversations for achievements by members of your network. This offers an opportunity to make a phone call or write a note to congratulate them and reconnect. Periodically skim through your address book, Rolodex, and business card files. Note those network members with whom you have not had contact in a while. Call or write to reconnect and share what each of you is currently doing.

Although it is a difficult step for some professionals to undertake, use your network to ask for needed information or expertise. We like to appear competent and confident in front of our colleagues and sometimes see asking for help as a sign of weakness. We are also afraid of imposing on our colleagues. Remember, though, that we all need assistance and information at one time or another. Ask for assistance if you need it; by doing so, you let your network members know that you depend on them just as they can depend on you. The more experienced we become, the more important this step may be. Others may see us as not needing any help when we have more experience or expertise than they have.

Remember to ask what you can do for the other members of the network. This step is frequently neglected. Even with the best active listening skills, you may not discover the needs of the members of your network, and they may be shy about asking for your assistance. By asking what you can do for them, you discover what they really want help with, take the pressure off them if they are unwilling to ask, and make your willingness to help apparent even if you cannot help at the time. But when you offer help, be realistic. Do not promise things you know you cannot do. If you are unsure of something, only promise to try. Be aware of time commitments, and do not overextend yourself. Realize that your credibility may suffer if you must later renege. Build your reputation on your integrity and credibility. If you are unable to do what you promised, get back in touch and explain what you were able to accomplish and why you could not do what you promised.

If you incorporate these steps into your networking process, information and assistance will be flowing both to and from you. Your network will become one of your most prized assets, and you will have made communication one of your master skills as a manager.

Summary

The effective manager understands the critical impor-tance of formal and informal communication to his immediate and long-term success. Essential to effective communication is understanding fundamental strategies for communicating at different levels of the organization, being aware of the effect of individual differences upon communication, and, of course, being a good listener.

SPECIAL ISSUE

THIS ITEM IS RESERVED

FOR ANOTHER READER

AND CAN ONLY BE

ISSUED FOR 7 DAYS

PLEASE RETURN VIA

THE BLACK BOOK BIN

4

Planning Strategically:
A Step-by-Step Guide

In many communities, there will be one or two health care providers that constantly seem to lead in the development of new services and new ways to deliver existing services. These market leaders then force competing providers to mimic them to remain competitive. What sets the innovators apart? How do they always seem to move so quickly from a management idea to implementation? While creativity is certainly a factor, it is only one reason. There are two. To realize creative management, innovators must be powerful planners. Planning is often given only passing consideration by many managers, who prefer to focus their energies on the more action-oriented components of their work. What exactly is planning? It is a systematic process that results in four accomplishments:

- Clear, measurable goals and objectives
- An infrastructure for analysis and forecasting change
- Strategies to achieve objectives in the current environment and under projected alternative environments
- A system for evaluating the effectiveness of management strategy

Each of these aspects is valuable to the manager and is used in successive planning steps.

Many health care managers question the practical value of planning. They correctly note that "everything is changing so fast" and complain that by the time they get a plan written, it is obsolete. In an environment as volatile as health care, solid planning is even more critical than in a more stable arena. By complaining about not being able to "get a plan written," managers pinpoint their problem. Planning is not a *document*; it is a continuous *process*. On occasion, planning may result in some form of physical evidence such as a strategic plan or budget, but this is not always necessary or desirable. This chapter will demonstrate the benefits of making planning a continuous part of a manager's job and review the elements of effective planning for health care managers. It will also provide practical tools to make planning manageable and rewarding.

Characteristics of Successful Planning

Nearly every manager in the hospital, nursing home, or any other provider can claim to conduct planning of some sort. But not nearly as many can claim to be successful planners. Although the specific protocol of successful planning will vary from organization to organization, and even from department to department, there are several critical attributes that all planning protocols share. Successful planning is appropriately scoped in time and level of specificity, proactive and reactive, data based, and internally and externally valid. Explanations of these characteristics follow.

Appropriate Scope

An appropriately scoped plan covers a span of time that is reasonable for the planner to project realistically. An appropriate hospital strategic plan will address a time frame of three to five years. (Some go longer, but as the pace of change increases, the span of strategic plans contracts.) An effective strategic plan also addresses the entire corporate system under the hospital; all major departments will have a stake in the effective strategic plan. By contrast, the departmental plan will be shorter in duration and more concrete in nature. It will provide specific objectives for about a year and supporting steps for the achieve-ment of those objectives. Typically, department plans for periods beyond a year are limited to a statement of intended goals that will support the corporate strategic plan. The plan does not provide more concrete guidance beyond this time frame be-cause its importance as a part of the overall strategic plan may increase or decrease depending upon changes in the environ-ment or senior management priorities. For example, in one large hospital (320 beds) in a community of 250,000 people and four hospitals, the strategic plan called for increasing the hospi-tal's role in neonatal and pediatric health care. One objective of that plan was to establish a Level III (critical care) neonatal nursery (to provide advanced care for the most critical health care needs). Based on this strategic goal, the engineering depart-ment established in its plan for one year to determine physical requirements for a thirty-bed nursery. After six months, however, the state government awarded a certificate of need authorizing development of the nursery to a competing hospital. This en-vironmental factor made it unnecessary for the department to complete even this first objective. For the department manager to have developed a detailed two- or three-year plan specifying how he would obtain materials and manage construction would have been a waste of time.

Proactive Approach

Plans often will effectively assess the likely developments in a local community's health care environment and set forth objectives and steps to maintain a hospital or department's position in response to those changes. For instance, given a projected drop in the number of patients in the community, a hospital may plan to decertify a certain number of beds. A powerful plan goes beyond anticipating what the environment will do to a department and organization. It becomes an en-vironmental force in its own right. To continue my example, a proactive plan that anticipated a reduction in patient census might examine local demographics and conclude that there is an opportunity to convert the beds that would otherwise have to be decertified. This conversion might be to an extended care facility or perhaps to a modern birthing center, complete with private, single room labor and delivery, homelike furniture, and value-added family services.

Data-Based Planning

While the intuition that comes with experience is a valuable aid in management decision making, it should be used as a back-up tool and employed only in the absence of data to support decisions. Nowhere is this more important than in planning. The future is challenging to predict accurately with empirical data. Without it, planning becomes little more than a roll of management dice — and managers win about as often as craps players do. Two categories of data are important to a manager. The first type is trend data, which track changes in information over a period of time. With these data, a manager can (after considering other information) quantify the extent of change that may occur in the future and subsequently how much change in resource allocation is needed. The second type is static data, which will provide a portrait of some element of management. These data are helpful for comparing department operations and resource allocation to other departments and to standards in health care. An example of a manager using trend data is the nursing service director who knows that she currently is providing 60,000 patient days of nursing per year and that for the past four years, this figure has been falling by an average of 1.2 percent per year. She also knows that another local hospital, which is closing soon, provides 40,000 patient days per year and that this number has been falling by an average of 6 percent per year. Given these figures, the nursing director can project her staffing needs under a variety of conditions. If her hospital will be assuming 30 percent of the closing hospital's patients, for example, she can project staffing needs. An example of static data use in planning would be the pharmacy manager who will be setting up a pharmacy in a newly opening hospital. By comparing pharmacy use data from hospitals in similar metropolitan areas and in similar hospitals, the pharmacy's director could develop initial resource requirements for her initial management plan.

Internal and External Validity

Internal validity of a plan refers to its *consistency* with the strategic mission and particular goals that it supports and its *feasibility* given the existing management environment in the department and the organization. If a radiology manager plans to develop magnetic resonance imaging (MRI) services over the next two years at a hospital, but the hospital's strategic direction is toward geriatric and outpatient care, MRI will likely be inconsistent with the strategic plan and hence internally invalid. A hospital that is building its capacity to support chronic disease is unlikely to be able to justify the costs of establishing an MRI. This expensive technology would likely demand use in an area with more patients to justify its cost. Even when a plan is consistent with superordinate organizational goals and missions, it must be internally valid in other ways as well. Among these are consistency with expectations of other managers, particularly senior managers in the provider, and financial feasibility.

External validity refers to the feasibility of a plan given the realities of the health care market at large. In the past, the scope of external validity was limited to consideration of other, possibly competing departments in the same provider or other providers in the same community. External validity was essentially a local concern. Increasingly, though, in the past decade, external validity of a plan has come to be influenced by regional and national forces, including vertically integrated delivery systems competing with a provider in certain service areas, revisions to federally reimbursable services by the Health Care Finance Administration, and national health care demographics. An example of the impact of the national scope of external influences on a manager's planning is well seen in the managed care marketplace. In many regions of the United States, local and regional providers who are offering or are contemplating such services as Health Maintenance Organizations, Preferred Provider Organizations, and Individual Provider Organizations must seriously consider the impact of potential competition from a well-organized, nationally focused system such as Kaiser-Permanente. Kaiser and others, once regionally based, have successfully penetrated markets in the Southwest, Northeast, and Midwest. Because of their size and organization, these systems have contributed to the failure or cancellation of similar plans by many local providers.

Benefits of Planning

A major hurdle in my work with clients on the issue of planning is a perception of many managers that they are already doing planning as a regular part of their job. If this is the case, they reason, why bother spending more time on the issue? Most managers do engage in some form of planninglike behavior. But truly powerful planning requires some degree of formal structure and a disciplined method of data gathering and analysis. This does not mean that one must become a statistician to be a successful planner, but the process does require organization, analysis, and ongoing attention.

If one brings this discipline to the process of planning, the rewards reaped are far greater than those obtained with a loosely structured, seat-of-the-pants plan. Among these rewards are the ability to forecast changes in key factors of your management environment. An effective planning system allows the manager to track data that can affect his management decisions. For example, by having information about the monthly trends in the population of inpatient chronic cardiopulmonary disease, a nursing manager would understand trends in this portion of the inpatient population. She would know that patient bed use for the respiratory and cardiopulmonary care units would increase as much as 45 percent from late October through March. Another reward of planning is greater precision in resource allocation. Following my example to its next logical step, the manager would be able to project her staffing needs for the respiratory and cardiopulmonary units and allocate accordingly to meet the increase in patient volume. She would also be able to project demand for special equipment, such as tracheostomy care supplies, ventilators, and electrocardiogram monitoring disposables. Even without understanding why this increase would likely occur, the manager would be prepared to anticipate its development. A third reward is cost savings as a result of preemptive and contingency planning. In my example, the manager would be able to save primarily payroll costs by anticipating the rise in chronic obstructive pulmonary disease, congestive heart failure, and patients with similar problems. By anticipating the change, she would staff the units that would care for these patients at higher levels, with additional staff coming from other care areas where patient populations might be projected to fall and with part-time support. The part-time support would provide basic nursing, which would free the regular unit staff to manage more complicated aspects of patient care. Part-time staff would also provide the manager with an appropriate response if a predicted influx of patients did not occur for whatever reason. Part-time employees are not guaranteed specific work hours or shifts and could be cut back if not needed.

Six Steps of Planning

Regardless of the specific planning procedures employed in any given organization, six steps must occur if planning is to be successful. These steps can be identified in successful planning of both formal, long-range planning and day-to-day planning that may never be documented. These steps are:

- Establish objectives.
- Define priority environmental parameters.
- Collect data to measure current environment.
- Forecast likely environmental developments.
- Develop strategies to achieve objectives.
- Evaluate strategies and objectives after implementation.

Although these steps are listed in sequence, they actually are

Figure 4.1. Steps in the Planning Process.

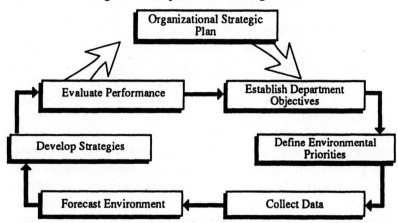

cyclical in nature, like any ongoing process. The success of each step depends upon the quality of management information in the previous step. The relationship between the planning steps and between department-level planning and strategic planning is demonstrated in Figure 4.1.

Establishing Department Objectives

The old saying, "If you don't know where you're going, it's easy to get there," applies well to many aspects of health care. Most health care managers readily see the importance of technical goals, but fewer see the relationship between planning goals and objectives and management success. An example of a technical process goal in health care is the indication for a particular type of therapy. For instance, the indication or objective for the use of aerosol bronchodilators is the relief of bronchospasm. It is crucial that managers have a clear understanding of both technical process and managerial objectives. It is no less important that those goals and objectives be concrete, measurable, and consistent. One reason it is so easy to see the specific objective of a clinical intervention is the immediacy of its effect. One knows (generally) if a bronchodilator has worked for a patient. Within minutes a patient will stop wheezing and start breathing clearly. Because the time elapsed between the setting of a management objective in a planning process and the assessment of that objective can be weeks or even months, the relationship between goals and outcomes can be less obvious to the manager. How can a manager set planning objectives to guide the development of strategy and form a basis for evaluating department performance? This is possible if objectives are demonstrably supporting one or more strategic priorities of the entire provider organization and are constructed for use as a management tool.

When beginning the planning process at a department level, a manager should first look to the organization's strategic plan and the objectives it cites as priorities. All department-level objectives in the provider organization should directly contribute to the successful accomplishment of at least one of the goals stated in the organization's strategic plan. The strategic plan for the organization is a long-range plan (typically three to seven years, with most spanning five years) that specifies global goals and objectives for the entire provider organization. The reason managers should develop their planning objectives to support strategic goals and objectives may seem obvious to many, but its importance is such that I will state it plainly. The organization's overall success is the greatest single determinant of many factors that are important to every employee. Among these factors are such fundamentals as staffing levels, budget size, and quality of care available. The strategic plan reflects the considered opinion of the CEO, the board, and senior managers about the business and service direction that presents the best opportunity to provide needed services to the community and remain in the best possible financial position. To succeed as a manager, one must often first consider the organization as a whole. The most effective way a manager can do this is to identify the priorities of the organization's leadership and then plan strategy that will support those priorities.

Strategic goals and objectives are so broad that they almost always cross departmental boundaries. They are also so broad that they defy precise quantitative targeting. A typical strategic goal might be "Become positioned as the region's preeminent gerontologic care provider." Now, this goal, while commendable, is not readily amenable to specific quantification. The more specific strategic objective that would support this goal might read "Increase market share for inpatient elder-care services by 25 percent in the next three years." The strategic objective is certainly measurable but only in the broadest sense. It does provide a foundation for department managers by communicating that gerontologic services are a priority for the organization. It also provides them with a target of a 25 percent increase in total market share, but even this is not very helpful in day-to-day management.

So how can a department manager use strategic goals and objectives as a starting point for developing planning objectives? Using the strategic priorities communicated in the plan, the manager can develop a draft of planning objectives designed to contribute specifically to one or more of the strategic objectives. The exact nature of the objectives drafted will vary depending on the services provided by the manager's department, but virtually all managers in the organization will find themselves able to contribute in some measurable way to the strategic success of the organization as a whole. For an example of how a strategic goal translates to a variety of departmental planning goals, see Figure 4.2. In this figure the strategic goal, "Become positioned as the region's preeminent gerontologic care provider," is successively refined and made more concrete. The first step in this process is to more precisely establish a strategic objective that will indicate whether the organization's overall goal is being achieved. In this example, this is done by establishing, at the level of senior executives, a strategic objective to "Increase market share for inpatient elder-care services by 25 percent in the next three years." To measure this, one needs to determine present market share and then reassess that share in three years. Finally, using the strategic objective as a starting point, department managers determine what specific things they can accomplish to help realize that objective.

There is a cautionary note to be added here about the process a manager uses to develop planning objectives. The process must ensure that it has the support of the administrator

or senior manager to whom the department manager reports
and the support of the supervisors and shift leaders in the
department. This will be discussed in greater detail later in this
chapter. Specific strategies for achieving this support can be
found in Chapter Six. Notice how different the respiratory care
objectives are from the nursing objectives and the marketing
objectives. Yet each objective, if accomplished, will directly contribute to the strategic goal.

What makes an effective objective? Focusing on four considerations when developing planning objectives will ensure
that they are precise and useful in guiding the planning process.
These considerations are the people involved, the outcome
expected, the parameters, and the extent of successful accomplishment. In this approach to developing objectives, the manager must clearly specify four elements:

1. People: Determining who is involved in completing
the objective will enhance accountability in meeting the objective. As health care moves toward vertical integration of services
for specific groups in the community, the people component of
planning objectives becomes more imperative than ever before.
Vertical integration frequently requires that several departments work together or at a minimum be consulted to successfully achieve plan objectives. An excellent example of this type
of interdisciplinary work is the establishment of home care
services. In such an effort, input and active ownership of plan
objectives must be obtained from nursing, respiratory care,
social services, and several other departments. In such complex
planning efforts, the manager must indicate which departments
will be responsible for which components of the plan.

2. Outcome: Planning objectives must specify the exact
outcome of the plan. This outcome may or may not be a fully
operational service or other improvement, but it should nonetheless be specified. There are several reasons for specifically
describing the outcome of the plan. It will facilitate input and
guidance on the plan from senior managers. It also helps ensure that there is a common understanding of expected
performance.

3. Parameters: In addition to indicating what will be

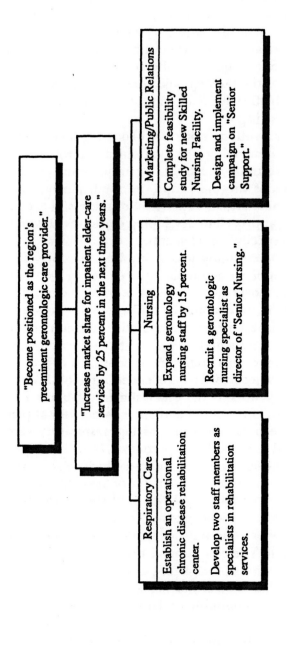

"Become positioned as the region's preeminent gerontologic care provider."

"Increase market share for inpatient elder-care services by 25 percent in the next three years."

Respiratory Care

Establish an operational chronic disease rehabilitation center.

Develop two staff members as specialists in rehabilitation services.

Nursing

Expand gerontology nursing staff by 15 percent.

Recruit a gerontologic nursing specialist as director of "Senior Nursing."

Marketing/Public Relations

Complete feasibility study for new Skilled Nursing Facility.

Design and implement campaign on "Senior Support."

accomplished and who will be responsible for accomplishing a plan, objectives must indicate the parameters or conditions under which the work can reasonably be expected to be accomplished. This also serves several purposes. One is to provide information for senior managers to react to and supply an opportunity for them to identify additional or heretofore unknown constraints upon a plan. Planning parameters address relevant variables associated with the project or service(s) planned. Typically this will include time requirements, personnel, interdepartmental support needed, projected cost data (if available), and administrative prerequisites. An example of the importance of planning parameters is well demonstrated in the case of a nursing manager who was strongly encouraged by the director of nursing (DON) to commit to developing a pre- and postoperative patient education and assessment service for cardiac surgery patients. This education was to be support service for a planned cardiovascular surgical unit at this hospital. When the nurse manager asked how necessary resources would be made available, he was told that those would "be taken care of." The plan, as the DON saw it, was to establish the services and formally request funds of the CEO, who was "staunchly behind" the development of a state-of-the-art cardiovascular care unit in the hospital. The nurse manager subsequently planned and committed to the development of the patient education service, which called for at-home preadmission education via videotape, preoperative education for patients and families, and a two-week postoperative home follow-up. The plan was accepted enthusiastically by the DON, the CEO, and the recently appointed chief of cardiovascular surgery. However, only the DON and the nurse manager knew about the DON's commitment of unbudgeted dollars to pay for the service. The CEO assumed that the nurse manager who had developed the plan for the service had also budgeted for the service.

4. Extent: All planning objectives should specify the extent of completion planned for a project or function. One might assume that any plan, whether for annual operation of a department or establishment of a new service, would naturally include implementation and evaluation. This is not always the case.

Special projects in particular are frequently limited to analyzing the feasibility of a concept promoted by a member of the medical staff or administration. Some plans only require evaluating several alternatives to accomplish a particular task and do not need to address other management concerns, such as staffing patterns, operational budgets, and quality control. For example, one midsized hospital recently decided to determine the best way to provide diagnostic laboratory services for physicians and their patients; at the time, an independent laboratory provided such services. All staff and equipment in the lab were provided by that contractor. Rather than ask the possibly biased lab manager to make the determination, a nursing manager and the laboratory medical director were given that task. In this case, the planning objective is to determine whether it is more feasible to continue contracting lab services or to establish internal lab support. The objective does not extend to planning lab services or developing a work plan to establish operations.

Defining Environmental Priorities

Conducting an environmental assessment is something traditionally associated with institutional strategic planning. Trends in health care management over the past decade are requiring that this activity also become a formal component of the department manager's planning. Among these trends are a reduction in the number of management layers between the CEO and the department manager and a growing appreciation for the intimate knowledge that department managers have about their customers. What is an environmental assessment? Why should a department manager concern herself with something as "esoteric" as an environmental assessment? Is not that what marketing and planning departments are for?

Internal and External Environmental Assessment. An environmental assessment allows a manager to define the elements of both internal and external environments that will impact the planning process. The internal environment consists of those components of the provider organization that are under the manager's control. Typically this is the performance of the department for which the manager is responsible. The internal environment does not refer to other departments in the organization. Those areas will have an impact on the planning process, but will be considered part of the external environment because they are outside of the manager's control. The external environment includes all other departments in the organization, plus the local, state, and even national forces that can influence plan design and execution.

The internal environmental analysis will enable the manager to determine, based upon past department performance, the likely impact of the plan upon current performance levels and which departmental components will play the biggest role in achieving the plan's objectives. Critical considerations for the manager in assessing the internal environment focus on three areas: capacity to support the plan, development needs, and physical needs.

The ability of a department to achieve plan objectives is especially important when a manager will roll out a new service to be provided by her department. The manager must assess the current work load of the department and determine how the plan will affect that work load. The likely impact of the plan on all other resources necessary for department operation must also be considered. These resources include budget, time, and materials needed for department operation. If there are any likely capacity issues, subsequent management strategy must address them.

After conducting a global analysis of departmental work capacity, the manager must assess the ability of the staff to perform in the general areas required by the objectives. If there is any question about the experience or preparation of staff, then management strategy must specifically address this issue. The most frequent saboteur of otherwise well-developed plans is the inability of staff to deliver because of inexperience. For example, I have seen many home health care programs stumble, falter, and even fail because managers failed to adequately assess the experience of their staffs in the provision of care in a home. The environment at home is very different from the totally equipped inpatient facility. Patients present many challenges seldom seen by the care giver in an institutional setting. These factors have an impact upon either developing existing staff or adding new staff to support the plan.

Finally, an assessment of the internal environment should include a preliminary assessment of whether the planned objectives will have an impact upon the existing physical environment. Will additional office, work, or storage space be needed? If so, the manager must identify these issues and develop strategy accordingly.

An assessment of the external environment enables the manager to gather five crucial types of information for making decisions:

- Preferences of customers
- Developments by competing providers in the manager's area of responsibility
- Physicians' opinions of and likely responses to new developments
- Current developments in the science or technology for which the manager is responsible and likely developments in the near future
- Current legal and political issues affecting the manager's area of responsibility and their likely resolution

Some of these areas of planning information may make perfect sense to many managers, but others may not, at first, seem relevant.

Customer Preferences. Customer preferences refers to the needs and wants of the people served by the manager's department. Now this may seem like a strange idea to nurses or physical therapists who see only their patients and turn sour faces at the word *customer*. It is, nonetheless, an issue in health care that will become more rather than less prominent in the foreseeable future. To be useful, a customer preference profile should be an ongoing effort in a department and contain data formally gathered periodically and informal observations and insights

Figure 4.3. Department Customers: First Breakdown.

Facilities	Nursing	Public Relations
• Nursing Staff	• Patients	• CEO

• Physicians
  -surgery
  -pediatrics
	• Physicians
	
	• Families
		• Department Managers
		
		• Patients

• Departments
  -intensive care unit
  -operating room
		• News Media

• Patients		

gathered in daily contact with staff, other departments, physicians, patients, and their families. Perhaps the greatest strength of the "management by walking around" philosophy is that it allows a manager to unobtrusively gather this and other management intelligence. A meaningful grouping of customers is any breakdown of the entire customer population that enables the manager to make decisions and plan services. These groups will differ from department to department. Figure 4.3 shows the difference between customer groups in three hospital departments.

This example shows only a preliminary specification of customer groupings. Most managers find that more meaningful information can be derived when more precise breakdowns are made. For example, rather than grouping all patients together, consider grouping them by similar needs and concerns. This may create groupings such as young families and chronic cardiovascular patients. Such groupings enable the manager to identify more quickly service needs and common customer preferences. Rather than belabor the issue of customer preferences, the manager should consult with in-house experts at tracking this demographically structured information. Marketing, planning, and public relations staff are generally experienced at this and will be able to assist managers.

Competitor Activity. Marketing and planning departments typically attend very closely to the plans (and rumors of plans) by competing providers with regard to new services, marketing campaigns, and other activity that might attract physicians and patients to their facilities. They are, however, often unable to gather information as quickly and accurately as needed because of the fiercely competitive nature of health care administration. The department manager, however, is in a uniquely well-suited position to gather useful information about activities in competing providers. This is because of the fraternization between staff and managers alike in many departments from many different providers. For example, nurses, therapists, and laboratory professionals in many communities often change employers but remain in the same community. Professional societies often bring together medical and allied health staff for education and social functions. Finally, allied health professionals in many communities were trained in the same schools, became friends, and went on to work for competing providers. All of these factors combine to make the alert department manager one of the best sources of information about competitors. This knowledge can serve the manager in planning for his department, and it can serve his career by contributing to institutional planning efforts. CEOs and marketing executives increasingly are realizing this fact and tapping department managers for this knowledge. Indeed, many corporate marketing services in hospitals today view their role as consulting with department managers on the best ways for managers to serve a marketing role.

Physicians' Opinions About New Developments. Despite the revolutionary change in American medicine in the past decade, one thing is constant. The most powerful figure in most providers is the attending physician who admits the most patients. The department manager is in closer daily contact with specific physician groups than any other manager in the organization. Senior managers have contact with key medical staff members, but this contact is not at the point of service — the clinical floor or medical records room. This means that the department manager has ready access to important information about likely medical staff support for plans. The manager also has the opportunity to develop plans that respond specifically to the needs of physician groups who are primary customers.

For example, through frequent formal and informal contact with anesthesia and pulmonary medicine departments, a respiratory care manager can gather information about physician requirements and preferences for postoperative intensive care support and rehabilitation services for chronically ill patients. With this information, the manager can plan in these areas with confidence that plans will meet the needs of one of the most important customer groups — physicians. Political realities of the provider organization and resource scarcity make this a crucial step in the planning process. Meeting the needs of physicians will facilitate their support of a manager's plan. This support often means the difference between administrative approval (and the funding that accompanies that approval) going to one plan or another proposal competing for administrative priority.

Current Technology. Senior managers in a provider organization should be expected to have only a general understanding of current technology in various medical and allied health professions. In most cases, managers at this level have several departments reporting to them, some or all of which are beyond their areas of technical expertise. These managers, however, must still make decisions about the acquisition, use, and disposal of equipment and protocol in these departments. It becomes the responsibility of the middle manager to constantly monitor developments in the technologies of their area. This responsibility can be only partially delegated to supervisors and staff.

Tracking and evaluating technology is paramount for clinical and nonclinical managers alike. Recent advances in food storage, transportation, and communications technology have come at a pace that is nearly as vigorous as that of clinical technology. And only the middle manager is at once linked to the practical use of technology and the decision makers in the organization who will approve its use. Senior executives depend on the middle manager to evaluate the use of this technology.

The quality of the manager's advice in this area can lead to tremendous advances in the quality of care and to great reductions in the cost of providing services. It can also lead to an executive's approval of an expensive, inefficient technology that will be obsolete in one or two years. There are many examples of this in contemporary health care management. One is the advent of nuclear magnetic resonance and its rapid obsolescence with technological refinements that created safer imaging with magnetic resonance imaging (MRI). Even after it became clear that MRI was a viable technology, middle managers were and continue to be critical trend monitors for senior executives. The middle manager, by monitoring industry and management technology closely, can often advise and cite examples of the alternatives to acquire the imaging technology most effectively. Rather than purchasing the expensive equipment outright, astute radiology managers can advise about other strategies for establishing the service — such as lease agreements with manufacturers and joint ventures with physician groups. This information is regularly available in journals, at conferences, and through peers of the radiology manager.

The use of ultrahigh frequency mechanical ventilation to treat patients unable to breathe under their own power provides another example of the need for managers to monitor and evaluate emerging technologies. In the early 1980s it was discovered that patients with pulmonary disease could be "safely" ventilated using very high air pressures (over fifty pounds per square inch) and very rapid breathing rates (well over sixty breaths per minute). This revolutionary technique also avoided many of the side effects of traditional mechanical ventilation and so was attractive to physicians and managers alike. Equipment manufacturers also loved the concept and quickly began producing these new ventilators. Today, after many providers invested in this technology, it has been found to have serious problems and is no longer in wide use. Only the midlevel manager in the respiratory care department or the cardiovascular service (product) line was in a position to evaluate both the technical feasibility and the management implications of the technology. Only she was capable of providing a recommendation that balanced management and health care concerns.

Current Legal and Political Issues. No environmental assessment should overlook the impact of political and legal developments that might affect a plan. In the past it would suffice for the department manager to have a general understanding of contemporary issues that were confined to his specific department. Today, however, the manager must also monitor state and national developments as well. These political and legal issues can affect virtually every aspect of the department, as well as its relationship with other organizational entities. While the nursing manager might not initially see a direct relationship between proposed changes to federal regulations covering Medicare reimbursement for home care and the operation of her inpatient nursing service, the impact could be dramatic. If those regulatory changes restrict the types of home care services that Medicare will pay for, home care companies will quickly make them unavailable. Then all patients who require those excluded services will be forced to get care through an extended care facility or a hospital.

State politics can also impact the middle manager directly and in many ways. In several states there are currently efforts to require certain allied health professionals, in addition to nurses, to be licensed. The potential ramifications of these efforts include increasing the quality of care provided by ensuring uniform practitioner competence, decreasing the quality of care by reducing the number of available practitioners and overworking them, and increasing the cost of operating affected departments by forcing higher pay for licensed professionals. The manager who does not attend to these developments will find his plans inadequate.

Data Gathering

Once a manager has defined the environmental issues most important to successfully achieving objectives, she needs evidence to allow her to predict the future internal and external environments. To plan for the future, managers must be able to predict it. Effective data gathering is essential to successful predictions.

Managers are generally most comfortable with data when they can be quantifiably gathered and statistically manipulated. There is something comforting about being able to present data with 99.4 percent certainty about their precision. Yet, in practice, managers make many key decisions in the absence of statistical support. They are not guessing when they make these decisions; they are relying on data that can be gathered, analyzed, and understood but not well quantified. A good example of this qualitative data is the information a manager gathers while in the cafeteria or when talking with trusted staff members or physicians. Another example of qualitative information is the letter from the irate patient, or the phone call to the administrator that praises the new birthing center.

Data gathering in the planning process must use reliable methods for gathering both relevant quantitative data and important qualitative data. There is generally abundant consultative help available from the staff specialists in organizations large enough to have staff management specialists. Some of these specialists and the general type of data-gathering support they can provide the middle manager are financial, marketing, and external.

The chief financial officer (CFO) or one of his staff can generally advise managers on the most effective methods for determining financial return on investment in a project or service, the projected costs and revenues associated with a plan, and the relative feasibility of alternatives available for funding the plan. Many managers do not take advantage of the specialized skills and abilities of the financial office in a consulting mode. This can generally work against the managers and plans they are sponsoring. If the CFO is consulted in the data-gathering and forecasting phases of planning, the manager will benefit by having his concerns noted and seeking his advice about how to surmount those issues. If the manager does not consult the CFO, senior managers certainly will ask him to evaluate financial feasibility of the plan after it has been submitted for administrative review.

Gathering and analyzing data about the external environment is what marketing professionals do on a daily basis. They can advise the manager about the most effective ways to gather reliable customer information from physicians, other hospital staff, and the community. Marketing professionals can assist the manager in designing data-gathering systems that are free from bias, interpreting data, and transforming them into useful decision-making information. Given their constant immersion in the external environment and the tracking of competitors as well as industry trends, marketing managers and vice presidents can also assist the manager in determining general market feasibility of any new services planned.

There are many sources of industry data available to the manager. Of these, many are also low or no cost for use. The marketing office of most providers will routinely have available the more helpful of these. The American Hospital Association is composed of many special-interest professional groups. These groups can be a wealth of information and subject-specific data. The American College of Healthcare Executives is a personal membership professional society whose sole mission is to research and educate members on contemporary management issues in health care. In addition to these two sources, virtually every allied health profession has a society that provides valuable information to the department manager.

In addition to these sources of planning data, the following list presents useful techniques for gathering data for both internal and external environmental analysis.

Customer Preferences and Physicians' Opinions

- Walk around the facility on a regular basis, and observe interactions between customers and your staff.
- Incorporate a discussion of current customer-related issues as a regular component of staff meetings.
- Establish an ongoing dialogue with staff, customers, and the managers of internal customers on a regular basis. Those

unaccustomed to this may at first need to actually "schedule" informal conversations—for example, by planning to stop by and see Sally Jones in Nursing and buy her a cup of coffee. This planning can be done on a personal calendar until it is routine.

- Periodically stop by patients' rooms and chat informally about their care. Focus on items that are well received and those that could be improved. Ask patients what they would like to see done to make their stay more pleasant.
- Conduct periodic formal meetings with managers of internal clients to assess the quality of service provided and any emerging needs. The provider's marketing department can facilitate this until a manager becomes comfortable with this process.
- Using the marketing department as consultants, conduct periodic customer satisfaction surveys with each major customer group.
- Maintain a marketing log documenting pertinent findings from the preceding activities. Documenting these findings allows each item to be considered in context with all others and ensures that customer focus is a managerial priority.

Competitor Activity

- Consult with marketing and planning staff, who routinely monitor competitors.
- Talk with staff members, who likely have friends employed at competing hospitals. Occasionally, managers are a bit uncertain about this suggestion. But there is nothing unethical about it. The information you may receive is already "on the grapevine."
- Attend local professional group meetings. Many groups meet monthly and provide an excellent opportunity to network with peers.
- Consult with attending staff. If your department is a clinical service, the medical director is an ideal choice. Generally, attending physicians practice at several providers in the community, so they come in contact with managers and medical staff in several organizations on a daily basis. One

approach is to ask the medical director's opinion of priorities for the department over the next year or two, based on patient service needs and what she is observing in providers elsewhere.

- Establish an ongoing relationship with academic programs in medicine and allied health. Clinical affiliation with teaching institutions provides a manager with formal and informal opportunities to come in contact with faculty and students who are frequently rotating between providers.

Technology

- Share the task of gathering information, but retain the responsibility for final analysis of the impact of technology and current practice.
- Maintain active membership and involvement in relevant professional organizations. If you are responsible for several departments, you may need to rely on access to journals.
- Assign staff members responsibility for regularly scanning particular areas of professional concern and reporting on emerging technologies at in-service education meetings. For example, one staff member might follow developments in cardiovascular pharmacology, while another covers pulmonary function assessment.
- Tap faculty at local medical and allied health schools to provide periodic updates in an educational setting.
- Monitor vendor wares closely, and arrange for demonstrations and clinical trials when possible.
- Arrange for everyone in the department to attend regional or national professional conferences. If budgetary support precludes paying for every staff member every year, then provide support for top performers on staff, but insist that they each attend different conferences. Attend at least one national conference per year yourself.

Political and Legal Trends

- Review professional journals monthly. These journals should include at least two from each of the following categories: relevant medical, allied health, or technical specialty, senior health care management (*Modern Healthcare*, *Healthcare Executive*, or one of many American Health Association journals and magazines), and business management (*Harvard Business Review*, for example).

• Arrange for periodic workshops on political and legal issues by a senior manager in the organization. This may seem unorthodox, but it will ensure that you understand which issues are organizational priorities and will sensitize your staff to the issues.

• Maintain active involvement in state and national professional organizations. These groups generally monitor and interpret political and legal developments affecting their members.

Forecasting Environmental Developments

Armed with an understanding of key issues in the management environment and current and historical data about those issues, a manager next needs to predict how that environment will change over the time of the plan. Accurate forecasting is essential to every plan. In the past, forecasting in health care was considered a luxury to be indulged in only for strategic plans that spanned many years. And then it was done only to a very broad degree of accuracy. As our industry has become more dynamic, and as services have become vertically integrated, and thus more interdependent, forecasting has become a powerful tool for middle managers as well. Forecasting allows a manager to predict the likely obsolescence of technology, significant changes in cost structure, and developments with customers and competitors.

At the strategic level, forecasting must address a broad range of issues, including federal reimbursement levels for care, medical staff composition, and state and national developments. For the middle manager, the focus is more narrowly defined. Department-level forecasting must focus upon predicting staffing composition and costs, processes and procedures in practice, and technology and its impact on staff time and operating costs.

Staffing Composition and Costs. Staffing-related planning for the manager seeks to answer several questions: How will the staff be structured — with generalists or specialists? What will be the cost of this staffing? What staff support systems will be used? Even within our specialty structured health care system, the manager must still determine whether it is best to have extensively cross-trained staff generalists, where any staff member can rotate through any job function, or whether the work requires specialization and extensive practice. An example of a generalist structure is a primary care nursing structure, where a single nurse cares for total patient needs. In a specialist model, a medication nurse delivers drugs to patients, an intravenous (IV) team establishes and maintains fluid lines, and so forth. In forecasting this staff use and structure, the manager must consider many issues, including the staff's response to one arrangement or another.

Generalization often requires cross training of job functions; this has received mixed reviews by professional staff in many areas of the country. If a structure will require interdisciplinary cross training, there are even more considerations. Not the least of these is "Is it legal?" For instance, in licensed professions, cross training is generally prohibited. An obvious example of this is the universal prohibition against a licensed practical nurse dispensing medications. At the time of this writing, New York State is contemplating the licensure of respiratory care professionals. In addition to delimiting educational qualifications for these care givers, pending legislation may preclude other allied health professionals from performing certain invasive and diagnostic procedures that they have been allowed to perform in the past.

Processes and Procedures in Practice. Protocols for patient care, driven by technological advances and scientific discoveries, are changing at a rapid pace. The department manager must predict how these changes will develop and how they will impact the operations of his department or the project being planned. The most visible example today of how changing protocols affect management planning is the rapid evolution of care protocols for people with AIDS. Just a few short years ago, AIDS patients were treated simply for the particular superinfection that was diagnosed. As more was learned about the syndrome, however, treatment protocols evolved rapidly, and today those protocols impact virtually every clinical and support department in a hospital. Many protocol developments affecting how a manager will plan are driven by the increased use of home care, outpatient clinics, and other alternative delivery systems. If dialysis patients will be using inpatient services less frequently, will the manager need to plan home support by her staff for those patients? Will the walk-in clinic be supported with existing staff, or will dedicated staff specially hired for the purpose provide more effective care? Will a single management serve both satellites and the main provider institution, or will there be separate managers?

Technology and Its Impact on Staff Time and Operating Costs. The manager must evaluate existing data about technology and determine how it will affect his plans. A few years ago, the latest development in IV therapy delivery systems was a preset dose. This manually operated system automatically delivered a prescribed flow rate of fluid to patients. The system was a vast improvement over unmetered systems, but it still required set-up time, reservoir priming, and frequent monitoring and adjustment because the system depended on a manually set wheel valve for operation. The valve was subject to movement if patients were ambulatory or disoriented and agitated. The advent of electronic infusion pumps drastically reduced set-up time, monitoring, and adjustment needed for IV therapy. This more reliable system, however, also increased the knowledge requirements for IV therapists and floor nurses alike.

Mechanical ventilation of patients is a process that changed almost overnight. In the recent past, if a patient needed mechanical ventilation, a therapist needed to spend twenty to thirty minutes literally assembling a ventilator with wrenches and then testing it for safety and precision. This was not an ideal patient care protocol, but the alternatives for the patient were worse. Once the patient was receiving care, a clinician needed to monitor the equipment constantly, as its performance varied with the patient's condition. Today, technology has not reduced the need for monitoring, but it has greatly reduced the time needed for the task and the frequency of clinician intervention to correct fluctuations in performance. This is the result of "on-board computers," which automatically sense patient status and adjust performance accordingly. The machines also monitor physiologic parameters continuously and record them for clinicians. This has reduced the time requirements for therapists, but has greatly increased what care givers need to know to understand and manage the technology.

These and other technical advances also affect the cost of operating a department. The mechanical ventilator that had to be assembled with a wrench cost about $4,200 per unit. New, computer-assisted models can cost as much as $18,000 per unit and require much more sophisticated in-house preventive maintenance. The manager must accurately predict what these developments will be and how they will affect his plans.

Given all of these factors, it can be difficult for a manager to predict precisely how the work environment will take shape. To increase the effectiveness of environmental analysis, managers must make data gathering and environmental monitoring a continual process rather than something done exclusively at the start of large projects or when it is time to develop an annual operating plan for a department. This can be done by developing data-tracking systems for each area of management concern. Tracking data and documenting significant developments as they develop provide the manager with information that will be more reliable than memory when it is needed for planning. These systems can be as simple as a paper filing system or as sophisticated as computerized data systems that store and analyze data for the manager.

Computer support of planning analysis also provides the manager with another powerful tool to improve the accuracy of forecasting. Using computers allows the manager to rapidly explore alternative scenarios that may develop. By manipulating cost data, work volumes, and other key variables, a manager can quickly see how they will impact a plan. Software systems to allow this modeling can be a simple spreadsheet or data-base program or a sophisticated (and generally expensive) project modeling system.

Many health care managers, whose children are growing up with personal computers, do not themselves tap the power of computers to enhance their management planning and decision making. In the past, this reluctance to embrace computers was supported by a logical argument about the complexity and relative cost of computers and the programs that run on them. The past four years have literally transformed the computer industry, however, and today even the least computer-friendly manager can easily use planning software more powerful than programs that run on some large mainframe computers. These programs will allow a manager to enter important information about a department, such as staffing costs and coverage. This information can be manipulated and evaluated and influence the manager's assumptions about the department.

For example, a manager might assume that the average daily treatment load for a staff of 10 therapists is 70. Using a department simulation model the manager can increase this work level to 120 and have the software calculate the impact of that change upon staffing requirements, personnel costs, and the actual distribution of staff over a period of time. By using the computer to determine the impact of a variety of possible scenarios, a manager is better able to anticipate possible developments that will affect her department and then plan contingency responses to each eventuality.

Managing Strategy Development

When planning objectives are developed, data collection is completed, and a thorough analysis of the management environment has been conducted, management strategy can be developed for accomplishing objectives. There are many different approaches to strategy development, but the two most prevalent are objective-based and resource-based development.

Objective-based strategy development is analogous to zero-based budget development. In zero-based budget development, one considers constraints to financial resources *after* determining what is required to accomplish a goal. In this model, all costs are determined initially by estimating actual projected costs. When this is done, if a budget is larger than available funds, the budget is analyzed, not for areas where there is "fat" but to identify alternatives to the elements listed in the initial plan. If this is unsuccessful, the objectives and scope of activities can be constrained.

Similarly, in management strategy development, objective-based development requires a manager to develop a critical path of events necessary to accomplish planning objectives. Once these events are defined, resource requirements are determined for each event. Finally, a management plan is established that ensures that the resources will be obtained and that events will occur on time and within budget. Objective-based strategy development is an ideal approach for any planning, but is critical when planning new projects for which there is little precedent in the organization.

An alternative to this approach is resource-based strategy development. Essentially, this model evaluates existing resources and then searches for ways to accomplish objectives within the constraints of those resources. This is similar to developing a budget by evaluating a previous year's budget, increasing it by an inflation factor, and then allocating money according to priorities. The advantage of this type of budgeting and strategy development is that it is more quickly accomplished. A disadvantage of this approach in a rapidly changing environment is that it tends to maintain a status quo rather than encourage new and innovative solutions needed for success.

The first part of strategy development requires a manager to determine what will be done, who will do it, and when it will happen. Depending upon the complexity of the plan and the certainty with which the manager can schedule resources, this part of the strategy can be as basic as a "to do" list distributed to the people who will work on the project or as complex as a series of Gantt charts detailing project phases and accompanied by a detailed work schedule. Rather than belabor the logic of how one determines what must be done, I will emphasize a set of heuristics, or rules of thumb, that will enable a manager to ensure that a strategy receives support from key people and then discuss several techniques for building and communicating a management strategy.

Use a Straw Man. Begin by drafting a tentative, preliminary, and otherwise qualified strategy that includes each major step in the project, what will be produced as a result of each step, who will be accountable for completing each step, and when each step should be completed. I stress qualifying the initial draft because its purpose is not to communicate what will be done but to solicit input from supervisors, other managers, and superiors about the draft plan. Creating a straw man that invites reaction and constructive criticism is a more effective approach to quickly getting the feedback a manager needs than simply approaching someone and asking, "So, Charlie, how do *you* think we should tackle this one — huh?" It also focuses the attention of various experts on those areas with which they are most familiar. In addition to tapping the collective wisdom of a variety of interested parties, this approach has a predictable side effect for the manager who develops the strategy. People who review and comment on a draft strategy are more likely to support its implementation than if they had not reviewed it prior to implementation.

This approach is very helpful for the manager in two planning situations. If the project is a complex interdisciplinary effort, it enables the manager to quickly plan for variables beyond her technical expertise. If the project is politically sensitive, a manager can help to build support from each of the political camps with a stake in the project. To be effective using the straw man approach, however, a manager must be confident enough to accept legitimate criticism and suggestions for improvement. She must also be prepared to listen to and reject ill-informed recommendations. Finally, the planning manager must defend her position as final strategist with accountability for success or failure of the plan.

Avoid Premature Budgeting. In an era of belt tightening, many health care managers overlook the strategic elements of a plan and focus prematurely upon associated costs of a plan. The middle manager who is responsible for planning either routine operations of a department or innovative new services will become painfully aware of this. It is not uncommon for senior managers, financial officers, physicians, or even board members to "stop by and chat" with a planning manager.

The intent of these "informal" discussions is to learn more about projected costs or to lobby for items in a plan. Often the manager involved will feel an obligation to "please" his sponsors by planning to keep costs to a minimum or to defend them against perceived detractors of a plan. This can result in an unrealistic cost model that is doomed to fall short of a necessary budget. Avoid projecting costs with certainty and committing to those cost estimates until a preliminary strategy is established.

An excellent example of this occurred in a midsized regional medical center (220 beds) in rural Kentucky. A department manager had recently completed an analysis of the center's practice of contracting diagnostic testing and medical interpretation of those tests to an independent laboratory and a private medical group. He concluded that the medical center could save $75,000 per year by providing all lab services through the hospital. An attending pathologist would become the medical director for lab services and would receive a "bonus" for ensuring accurate clinical interpretations of lab work as part of his routine duties. The manager began receiving early morning visits from an attending nephrologist, who just stopped by to chat about mutual hobbies, hospital gossip, and such and have a cup of coffee. Over a few weeks, the nephrologist, who was also a partner in the private medical group providing the existing services, learned details of the plan and approached a friend of his who was an influential member of the board of directors. Although hospital boards typically restrict their activities to issues of institutional policy and governance, they do occasionally address significant operational issues. This board prevented the implementation of the manager's plan. The rationale was that the two years necessary to recoup the initial cost of equipment was too long a time to wait for the plan to "save any real money."

Tools to Develop and Communicate Strategy. An effective plan is much more than the document that communicates strategy and provides management information. People, effort, and resources make an idea reality. Yet, without appropriate documentation, a plan can rarely be successful. The plan documentation is the key to many essential events:

- Obtaining senior management support
- Evaluating strategy components and alternatives
- Getting access to people needed for a project
- Keeping project and staff members focused on task (particularly important on large long-term projects)
- Maintaining management decision making and control

What are the essential documents required for effective planning? To ensure that a plan is fairly evaluated and, if implemented, successful, every plan should include documentation of these components: plan objectives and rationale, environmental factors, and strategy.

Plan objectives should be clearly stated and expressed from the perspective of the plan's impact upon patient care, customer service, financial contribution, or strategic value of the plan to the provider. For example, consider a plan to revamp a communication system. An example of an inadequate objective would be "to modernize telephone, PBX, and paging systems." This may reflect what will be done, but it does not explain the reason it is being done. A more persuasive and accurate objective would be "to improve effectiveness of electronic communications by reducing lost pages, delayed PBX transmissions, and telephone users' reliance on switchboard operators."

The rationale section of plan documentation will explain the business or patient care needs that will be met by implementing the plan. This component of a plan will justify the plan to administrators who must approve it. The rationale should include an explanation of the strategic goals supported by the plan, and it should cite evidence to support the need for the plan. This explanation should effectively circumvent the "if it ain't broke, don't fix it" response that managers' plans occasionally receive. Cite as many of the salient reasons for implementing the plan as possible. Building on the objective of "improving electronic communications," one rationale might include this statement: "This plan will help realize the strategic goals of asserting our position as the most consumer-responsive provider in the metropolitan area. In a recent survey of county users of our services, 20 percent of all respondents cited delays in contacting physicians and hospital staff as a negative aspect of their experience with our institution. This plan will effectively eliminate that 20 percent opinion and enhance internal communication of administrative and emergency medical information."

A preliminary plan document should also include a summary of pertinent environmental factors contributing to the need for the plan. This should address each environmental area analyzed. A useful format for this is a brief summary of each significant finding, followed by specific evidence supporting that summary. Where possible, that evidence should be expressed quantitatively and supported by qualitative evidence. Direct quotes and paraphrases by people affected by a problem are particularly powerful for planning efforts directed to establishing or expanding services. After presenting a description of the current environment that will be improved by the plan, the planning manager, where possible, should describe in global terms the environment envisioned after the plan is successfully implemented. This should be done in general terms only and should speak to visible changes in management or operational efficiency. This component will enable administrators and potential implementors of the plan to envision its benefits.

Clear explanation of how a plan will be achieved — its strategy — is vital both to gaining acceptance for the plan and for guiding its implementation once approved. The strategy must be presented to administrative personnel and other gatekeepers at a high level initially and must address each of the components described in the section on strategy. When approved, either as submitted or as amended by administrative superiors, this component of plan documentation will then be elaborated into operationally precise work plans. For administrative approval and for periodic status updates, the following general format is usually effective:

- Project overview chart summary (Critical Path Method chart or Gantt chart presentations are generally useful.)
- List of achievements and due dates
- Labor requirements list, spread over project phases
- Estimated budget

A list of what will be produced is useful to administrative staff as a bottom-line picture of what can be expected as tangible evidence of progress with the plan. It can also enable them to evaluate the plan's comprehensiveness. Labor requirements allow administrative staff and any other managers involved in the plan to evaluate the feasibility of a strategy within time and work-load constraints. An estimated budget will provide a map for assisting cash flow and total funding requirements; few plans are approved without reasonable budget planning.

Planning with People. To this point, I have presented a walk-through of the critical components of planning and provided advice based on current management literature and empirical observation of dozens of organizations. This information will provide a framework for planning, but alone it will not guarantee successful management planning. The analytical and procedural components of planning are like the anatomy of the body. Having the proper structure is essential to effective function, but success requires a healthy physiology. The physiology of planning is the manager's ability to achieve support from administrative staff, physicians (where appropriate), other managers, and staff. Several other chapters of this book address these issues in detail, including Chapters Three and Six.

5

❧

Managing Projects:
Primary Principles and Effective Tools

The most dramatic changes in American health care are occurring in two areas: (1) the technology used to deliver care and (2) how services are packaged for delivery to customers. The most significant of these changes have been a result of project teams. This chapter addresses the important differences between effective project management and department, or functional, management. Today's health care manager must be adept at managing interdepartmental and even interinstitutional project teams. This is a departure from days past when most projects requiring coordination and cooperation from several departments were led by an administrative officer or an external consultant. Because of this expanded leadership expectation for the health care manager, effective strategies for project administration, project team leadership, and problem solving are also presented in this chapter.

Technology has improved constantly since the dawn of health care. But why is it now moving at such a rapid pace? This growth is possible because experts from very different areas of specialization are increasingly being brought together to work on specific projects. These projects allow cooperation and dialogue between formerly isolated specialists. This dialogue serves to cross-fertilize the creativity of all people involved in the project. Once the project is completed, experts are free to return to their traditional roles as specialists dedicated to work in their discipline—until it is time again to share their expertise with colleagues in other technical disciplines on yet another project.

The development of health care service lines for specific consumer market segments also requires the use of interdisciplinary teams of technical specialists. For example, the development of home health care services for the chronically ill would be best accomplished by a team of people, including social services, nursing, cardiopulmonary care, pharmacy, and physician representatives. Depending on the scope of services to be offered, additional expertise from facilities and physical therapy might also be needed. To sell the service to clients, expertise from the marketing and sales fields would also be helpful.

The management of such diverse teams of independent professionals presents a special challenge to the health care manager. Project team management is as different from administrative management of a department as night is from day, and the effective health care manager must be adept at both.

Project Team Management Versus Department Management

Regardless of whether a manager is handling a 60-bed nursing home or a 300-bed medical center, the process of project management requires a core of essential skills. These skills allow the manager to plan and make decisions about people's schedules and activities, resource acquisition and use, customer satisfaction, and the budget. This may seem similar to traditional department management, but the unique factors associated with a project's life cycle, the temporary nature of a project team, and other factors create special challenges.

None of this structure exists at the start of an interdisciplinary project. A project team is formed precisely because a need has been identified and no existing structure in the organization meets that need. The team is temporary and links people who do not usually work together and likely share nei-

Table 5.1. Differences in Department and Project Management.

Function	Department Management	Project Management
Planning	Repetitive with annual, monthly, weekly, and daily issues that are similar from cycle to cycle.	Single cycle of planning, broken into discrete phases.
Communication	Clearly defined channels which emphasize chain of command and adherence to procedure.	Must be more rapid, relies on both formal and informal channels. Meetings are more frequent.
Leadership	Generally hierarchical, multiple layers of administration.	More streamlined; requires advocacy rather than administration for leadership.
Roles and responsibilities	Clearly defined, supported by position descriptions, formal policy, and procedure documentation. Social pecking order determined by job.	Must be defined at the start of project and redefined as project progresses.

ther a common reporting relationship nor similar professional backgrounds. This disparity of formal reporting relationships and multiple professional identities combined with the transient nature of project work create unique challenges to effective leadership of project teams. Table 5.1 compares the critical differences between project team management and department management.

Project Planning and Organization

One of the most important aspects in effective project management is the organization and planning that must be done prior to even meeting with project team members. And with few exceptions, the greatest challenge to the manager of an interdisciplinary health care project is organizing to supervise effectively the activities of very autonomous groups of technical specialists who must work together on a project team. If not planned carefully and organized strategically, such projects at their best will plod along plagued by conflicts in professional opinions, differing political agendas of competing depart-ments, and the politics of life in a medical organization. At their worst, projects organized and planned poorly can be disastrous for the career of the project manager and the competitive posi-tion of the provider organization.

Avoiding Plodding Projects

If the project that plods along ever completes its assigned mission, the project team's recommendations will be obsolete as soon as (if not before) they are actually delivered. The results of this plodding are all disastrous. First, the project team's impact on the health care organization will at best be none. More likely, the failure of a project team to deliver on time will hinder the competitive advantage of the hospital or nursing home by miss-ing out on a precious window of opportunity in time. This window is a time when the organization can act to improve its effectiveness or market position with a particular project before competitors begin similar efforts. You will soon see a sad ex-ample of how a plodding project team cost one hospital the acquisition of a service line badly needed in its community. But how do you know a plodding project when you see one?

Three typical indicators of a project that plods along through inappropriate organization follow:

1. No one on the project team can tell you precisely which piece of the project is his. This is often the result of a very small scope of responsibility for many or all project team members, which destroys personal responsibility for the completion of any aspect of the project. This lack of identity also has a demoralizing effect upon the team members, who quickly feel like cogs of wheels.
2. Routine operating decisions take forever to accomplish. This slowness is often the result of too many levels of man-

agement on the project team, creating endless levels of approval for each step in project completion and delaying decisions.

3. A project team has advisory or administrative direction from more than one body. This multiple direction slows decision making and resource acquisition considerably. Perhaps more ominous is that this also creates an environment ripe for political gamesmanship between external bodies responsible for direction or advice to the project manager.

One project team that suffered from these problems was headed by a new administrative manager for a hospital attempting to get approval from the state of Illinois for a neonatal intensive care nursery. Acquisition of the nursery was important for the hospital for several reasons. Among them were the continued affiliation of a medical group of two prominent neonatologists and a pediatric cardiologist who were responsible for large research grants being awarded to the hospital. The hospital was one of three in the area petitioning the state for approval of the intensive care nursery. Because of the importance of the project, the hospital's anesthesia and surgery groups, administration, nursing, respiratory care, radiology, and laboratory departments all wanted to be involved in the design and planning of services for the nursery. The number of independent players who became active in the project was so large that communications and roles quickly became problematic. At the core of the difficulty was a lack of an organizational structure that would provide for input from each of these areas and yet limit the decision-making power to a manageably small number of players. While this provider's project team was waiting for approval from virtually every department involved on nearly all design and administrative issues in the project, the other two hospitals completed the entire application process eight and seven weeks before the application deadline.

When the deadline for proposal submission arrived, the plodding provider submitted a request for a deadline extension, which was rejected. The state's position was that there clearly must have been adequate time for preparation because they had received two applications long ago.

Organizing to Avoid Plodding Projects: Matrix Management Modifications

One popular approach to avoiding plodding projects is to use an organizational structure where project management functions are split into two components. In this structure, labeled *matrix* for the unusual organization chart it produces, there are two managerial roles that affect project staffing and project team management. The first managerial role, or function as it is often called, assumes responsibility for managing the production of one or more components of the project while staffing and the quality interests of various professionals are assumed by a second function.

The project production manager, referred to generically as a line manager, is responsible for satisfaction of the project customer, when the customer is the end user of the project's work. The line manager is the inside manager with regard to project completion. The manager in this project role is referred to as the project manager because of her intimate involvement with both day-to-day and long-range project planning and team leadership.

The second management function is responsible for managing the staffing and administration of the project. This staff management function essentially serves as the outside manager for the project and controls staff availability for project tasks and administrative communications with the provider organization and any other independent groups with input to the project. Because project teams are often composed of staff from several areas in an organization who lend their talent for the duration needed, there may actually be several different staff managers associated with a project. Each of these staff managers would coordinate with the project manager to provide individuals from their area to the project team on a temporary basis. For example, in the project shown in Figure 5.1, there may be a staff manager in neonatology, anesthesia, surgery, and nursing, all of whom will make some of their staff available to the project manager for project team work. Each of these managers would have a similar role in the project: suppliers of talent.

These project management functions can be compared to the management of a commuter train. In this analogy, the train engineer is the line manager for the project, controlling when the train leaves, how fast it travels, and when it stops. The conductor of the train is the staff manager, ensuring that passengers are accommodated and seated before the train's departure. The conductor, like the staff manager, makes the ultimate call as to whether a particular group of passengers really wants to board the train or whether they are waiting for another train.

In my example of the neonatal intensive care nursery, there was no delineation of these line and staff functions. If there had been such coordination, the project manager would have been free to control the operation of the project. Another role would have been established to assess the needs and interests of all physicians and departments involved, schedule staffing participation in the project, and define the parameters of that participation. This staff manager would also determine when and where problems with staffing and professional standards slowed the project and resolve such problems.

In large projects, this dual management function is divided even further, with staff management contacts allocated for each area of the organization involved in the project. While there will only be one line manager for a project, there may be several staff managers, each assigned from one of the areas of the provider organization. If this organization were applied to the ill-fated nursery project cited earlier, it might look like Figure 5.1.

This is a classic matrix organization. Each of the staff areas assigns a manager to plan with the project (line) manager the staffing requirements and administrative issues of the project. The project manager is responsible for conducting the development of the project's objectives, quality assurance, and day-to-day operations. In the example cited, the project team's overall aim is a petition to the state that contains all of the information necessary to obtain approval for the nursery. This

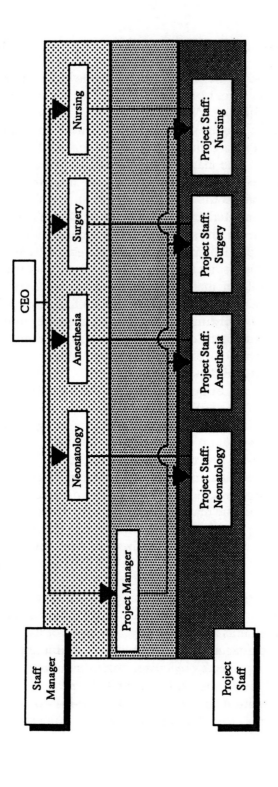

means that the project manager must determine what people are needed from each of the staff areas and what the staff from those areas will do if assigned to the project. In this way, each team member brings some special expertise that will result in the development of a specific objective.

Why use a matrix structure for projects where many different allied health and medical professions must work side by side? This organization allows the project manager to retain control of the critical time frames that often accompany a project and the direct responsibility and authority for ensuring the quality of the project team's work. At the same time, staff managers are effectively able to manage the staffing of multiple different activities and to act as advocates to ensure that the high standards of their department or profession are reflected in the project. The benefits of matrix approaches to project organization are considerable. Matrix management, however, is not a manager's panacea.

One aspect of matrix management that is disconcerting to many health care managers is that it appears to violate one of the cardinal rules of successful work — that is, each worker should have only one supervisor. In a pure matrix organization, staff managers retain responsibility for the ongoing administration of staff members assigned to the project. They also assume responsibility for developing the staff members assigned to the project. Now, to make this issue even more frightening to traditional health care managers, staff managers frequently assign staff to a project on a rotating basis. It is the staff manager's responsibility to standardize work procedures of staff on the project as much as possible. This is the only way to accommodate staff rotation and communication effectively. The project manager's responsibility is to determine how many staff will be needed from each area and the scope of their jobs and to manage their day-to-day performance. In other words, project staff report to a staff manager for scheduling and work assignments, but when assigned to a project they report to the project manager for project task assignments. The project manager is then responsible for evaluating the quality of work on project tasks.

This structure is extremely effective for managing the needs of client groups and the work-flow demands of a project's work schedule, but it definitely carries with it a high potential for creating conflict between line and staff managers. These tensions arise over conflicting priorities, poor communication, or changing agendas for each of the managers during the course of the project. The common aspect of nearly all of these conflicts is that they are played out at the staff level, with project staff being given conflicting requests, incompatible directions, and occasional ulcers. None of these things are conducive to a successful project.

The only effective way to avoid or manage these conflicts is through mature management on the part of both line and staff project managers. When problems arise in a matrix system, they are only effectively resolved through an informal system of communication and honest negotiations between the line and staff managers. Formal authority and politicking, two other often used management tools, are ineffective in a matrix system.

So what does a project manager do if matrix management is too avant garde for present purposes? It is admittedly fraught with risks of communication problems and power struggles. Although there is no one right answer to this question, several alternatives have proven effective, given the size and political sensitivity of any given project. Smaller projects, involving only two or three support areas and only one medical specialty, can benefit from collapsing the number of people who serve in staff management functions. This reduction involves having a single manager serve the staff function for two or more support areas. For example, one manager might be the staff manager for all of the ancillary services involved in a project. Mid- to large-sized projects can sometimes be managed more effectively in a health care organization if the scope of line responsibility is divided between two project managers who report directly to the CEO or most senior administrative officer responsible for the project. This limits the ratio of staff managers to line managers to a workable level, while retaining direct accountability for project deliverables.

Regardless of project size, the benefits of matrix management are better achieved while minimizing its risks by careful control of the communication system between line and staff managers. Project and staff managers should have regularly scheduled meetings on a formal basis, in addition to ongoing, informal meetings to discuss relevant planning and management issues. In addition, however, a second structure for formal communication should be established, in which all staff managers supporting a project manager meet with the project manager for a status briefing and planning future project needs. The value of this tiered system of formal communications is twofold. It allows individuals to discuss issues and concerns of importance in the privacy of a manager's office. It also brings many forgotten or hidden agenda items to the attention of the entire project team in an all-management staff forum, forcing the management of any inconvenient issues before they become major problems.

Seven Steps of Project Management

In management training, be it health care or more traditionally defined businesses, the function of management is to govern a diverse group of personalities to ensure their conformance to prescribed standards of work performance. This general approach is nowhere more inappropriate than in the management of projects for health care providers. In the environment of most provider organizations, project team members are working precisely because of, not in spite of, the differences between themselves and the people working with them. To be sure, while the interests and concerns of a physician and a plant engineer differ, they both want the new wing to be built in time and within budget. (The physician, as one of his agenda items, wants the wing to contain more office space, while the engineer wants to use low-maintenance materials.)

Effective project management requires the manager to define and redefine the common agenda of all parties involved in the project and to focus their energies toward the achievement of that common agenda. The project manager is not a governor so much as he is an enabler of staff achievement of common goals. The remainder of this chapter will focus on what that process entails and will provide practical tools and techniques for project managers.

Project management is an iterative process. It consists of repeating the same seven steps at progressively more refined levels of detail from the time project goals have been defined until the project has been implemented and evaluated. The seven steps of project management follow:

1. *Definition of project objectives.* This step allows the manager to clarify precisely what the client expects of the project. Most health care projects will have multiple clients, representing administrative, medical, and perhaps even public concerns. By defining the expected outcomes of the project first, the manager and the client together ensure that the project will proceed in the appropriate direction.

2. *Organize key project players.* With the goals defined, the project manager and the client will have a sense of what areas of the provider organization need to be involved. Tap these areas as a source of technical advice and staff management for the project.

3. *Planning.* Planning for a project involves many of the elements of planning the management of a department. Two critical differences between project planning and the more administratively stable functions of a department are in the time frame available to the manager and the degree of specificity required in planning at all stages of the project.

4. *Communicating.* No function is more crucial to the success of a project than effective communication of both plans and performance expectations. A poor plan can be improved, even in a short time frame, if it is completely communicated to the people affected by the plan. The feedback the manager receives from these people will provide for this improvement. But even the most brilliant plans for project execution need comprehensive communication starting with the project manager.

5. *Surveying.* Surveying involves the traditional processes of monitoring and assessment, but its purpose is not to judge

the worth of any idea, process, or person's performance in a project. Its purpose is to determine whether any particular facet of the project is performing consistent with the needs of the project. If it is, then it should be examined to determine what can be learned from it that may be generalized and used in other aspects of the project. If it is not consistent with the project's needs, then it must be surveyed to determine how to guide or change it to best meet the project's goals.

6. *Coaching.* Coaching analyzes human behavior and provides corrective and supportive feedback to guide that behavior to move in a desirable direction — in this case, the achievement of the project's goals. This function of project management must be served at two levels. Coaching obviously involves interaction between the project manager and project staff. What is often less apparent, however, is the coaching a project manager must do with staff managers and, in many cases, external personnel, such as physicians and board members, to influence their behavior for the achievement of the project's goals. For more on coaching, see Lombardi (1988).

7. *Revising.* Revising is the modification of current project plans to achieve the project's goals in the necessary time and resource constraints. Revising is to project management what adjusting a rudder is to sailing a boat. If after planning, communicating, surveying, and coaching a project team once, a manager has achieved her project goals, then the project was not complex enough to merit the effort of organizing a team. Much more often, however, a manager finds that even after solid plans have been made and communicated, they often need to be adjusted to accommodate unforeseen events, changes in deadlines, or loss of anticipated resources.

Definition of Project Objectives

Classic treatments of project management begin the process with defining the problem to be solved by the project. In practical instances, though, this step is often initiated by a board or administrative definition of the problem, and statement of goals related to that problem. In most health care projects, the problem is defined pragmatically as the refinement of general goals until they are concrete objectives.

The key issue at this point of project management is to achieve consensus from the most senior administrative, medical, allied health, and support personnel who will use the results of the project. The most important issues that all clients must agree on are the project's specific objectives, what will be needed to meet those objectives, and the main indicators that will be used to assess the project's success. There will always be room for differences of opinion regarding the methods used to achieve the goals of the project, but about these core issues there must be complete agreement.

Consensus is best obtained through a process where the manager accumulates information from clients one at a time and then resolves issues in a group setting. After interviewing individual clients to learn their expectations for the project, the manager must analyze their expectations and identify areas where there are differences in understanding the nature or scope of the project or potential conflicts in expectations for the project's outcomes. Once these areas are identified, the project manager is responsible for meeting with all of the parties together to communicate these outstanding issues and to reach consensus. One of the most effective methods for reaching agreement is the use of a modified nominal group technique. This process repeats a cycle of issue identification, clarification, and weighting, with each repetition narrowing and refining common priorities for a group. Many texts on group behavior provide detailed guidance on the use of the nominal group process; two that I recommend are *Introduction to Qualitative Methods* by Bogden and Taylor (1975) and *Qualitative and Quantitative Methods in Evaluation* by Cook and Reichardt (1979).

Organizing Key Project Players

Once the specific outcomes of the project are agreed on, it is time to build the core of the project leadership. The project manager must determine which areas of the hospital will be tapped for expertise, identify who will serve as staff managers for those areas, and orient them to the project and their roles in its success. Key outcomes of this important step are a project organization chart and a team of managers who understand the project's goals and are willing to support their achievement. In an environment as traditionally hierarchical and composed of autonomous professionals as health care, this can be a tricky thing to accomplish. Yet precisely because of this environment, establishing a clear structure for project personnel is imperative.

There are no magic pills to give to staff managers to infuse them with a desire to cooperate and support a project. What will go far in organizing a project team, however, is to structure the team to allow each manager the greatest possible control over the means she uses to manage her piece of the project. The structure of the project team should be limited to the following areas:

- A clear definition of the roles and responsibilities of each key project leader.
- A flat organization with the smallest possible number of managerial layers. Provide each project team member with a chart of the organization.
- An explicit communication protocol. As with the organization chart, this should be in writing and distributed to appropriate project team members before the project starts. This protocol should address administrative communications within the project team and between the team and the rest of the organization.

To the extent feasible, the project manager should allow the project's staff managers to participate in the development of project administration and communication protocol. In this way, each staff manager will be more likely to support the organization and management practices of the project.

Planning the Project

Planning enables the manager to acquire and use the resources (human, capital, and budget) needed to complete a project. Failure to plan removes this ability; when this happens the manager may as well wear a rubber coat and red helmet, because she is no longer a manager but a firefighter.

Planning the success of the project requires that the manager take given project goals and determine what resources will be needed, when, and with what effort, to accomplish those goals within existing time, money, information, and political constraints. I do not include the availability of labor among these constraints because in the absence of in-house staff availability, a lack of personnel can readily be subsumed within the category of budget constraints. The rationale for effective planning is older than the process of management. Indeed, the process of planning is to project management as the AAA "TripTik" is to vacation travel. It provides an overview of what routes or procedures must be followed, what milestones or landmarks one can expect at key times, and what specific step is next.

Planning is also like travel in that it is easier to do in general than in specifics. It is a simple matter to determine that if you are in New York and plan to go to Florida, you must travel south. So too, it is relatively simple to plan that to build a new women's health care clinic, you will likely need the input of Ob-Gyn specialists and pediatricians. From there, though, planning both a journey and a project becomes trickier.

The Goals of Planning. The goal of planning is to communicate to all concerned parties four crucial pieces of information they will need to contribute to its completion: the events that must take place (and the time frame for each event), the milestones completed (intermediate measures of project completion), the personnel requirements and time schedule for them, and the cost of all three prior elements. These costs are expressed in two different forms. The first is the actual cash outlay expended by the project's organization. An example of a hard cost is the purchase of new equipment to support a project. The second is the real cost to the organization, which includes both cash outlay and overhead or sunk costs, such as the cost of time for existing organizational staff to work on a project.

Planning Events: The Project Activity Map. While every journey begins with a single step, that step is preceded by reading a map, to make sure that you are on the right road. As the leader of the project, the manager must create the map that will guide the entire team from start to successful completion.

Making a project activity map (PAM) requires laying out each process that must occur in sequence for a project to succeed. Two facets of activity planning make it a bit trickier than it might initially appear. First, some project steps are sequence dependent. Certain steps must happen first to enable the success of subsequent project components. Certain other steps can happen at almost any step in the project, so long as they are completed before the entire project is unveiled. Second, some project steps can be sequenced only after input from specialists. This is because only the specialists who will be involved in those steps can determine what is prerequisite to their work.

One of the best ways to build and communicate a PAM is by using a chart such as the one shown in Figure 5.2. This PAM shows where each project step occurs in relation to others and quickly communicates all of the essential information of the activity map:

- Earliest possible start date for each step—the earliest point at which resources will be available for the project.
- Latest possible start date—the latest point at which a given project component can begin and still allow subsequent project phases to be completed on time.
- Earliest possible finish date for each step—the earliest point at which a step can be completed, assuming that its earliest start date was met and that all events occurred on time (usually a project manager's fantasy).
- Latest possible finish date—the latest point at which a given project component can end and still allow subsequent project phases to be completed on time.
- Critical pathway—the sequence of events that must occur for project success. All of the events in the critical pathway must occur in the order planned. The critical pathway ac-

tivities in a PAM are sequenced from left to right in a straight
line. Activities that can be completed concurrently with
other steps can be listed below or above these steps.

- Milestone activities—key actions producing a major objective of the project. For example, a project to establish a
  comprehensive elder-care facility could have as milestones
  the acquiring of land, obtaining a zoning permit, approving
  architectural plans, and opening the facility. Milestones are
  indicated with a different shape (often a rounded box) from
  other project activities. They measure progress and provide
  feedback to the project team.

How do you build a PAM if you are managing a technical
project where, to be honest, you do not have the foggiest idea of
how long it will take to, say, reprogram the financial accounting
computer to accept entries from a clinic you are planning to
buy? You can use an iterative approach to activity planning.
Develop a first draft of the necessary activities for the entire
project, along with the critical information outlined earlier.
Next, validate your plan by asking staff managers to review the
feasibility and completeness of both the sequence and time
requirements for each assigned phase. After all staff managers
have reviewed the draft plan, there will be feedback about miss-
ing steps, the amount of time needed for each step, and the
sequence of steps. With this feedback, the PAM can be revised
and reviewed until it represents a realistic plan of action.

Planning Project Resources. With the PAM as a guide, the
next step in planning the project is to develop detailed estimates
of the resources needed to complete each activity in the necessary time frame. For each box on the PAM, the project manager
must estimate the number and type of human resources needed,
the time required for the step by each person assigned, the
equipment and space needed by the project staff, and the cost
(including direct capital outlay for equipment, actual dollars to
be spent on any external services such as printing or consulting,
and the payroll cost for the project staff).

A powerful tool to plan and track the resources needed

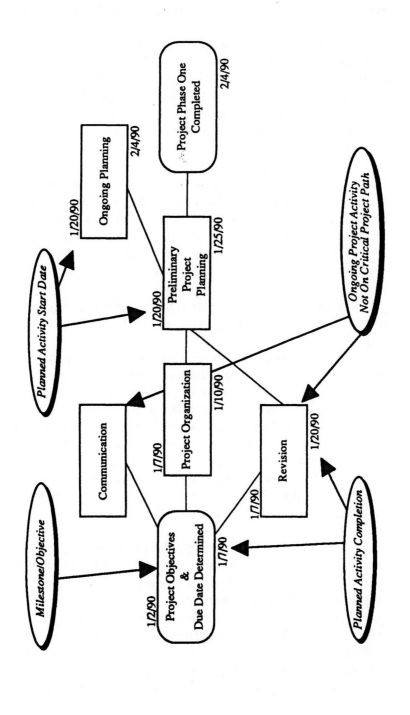

for a project is a Gantt chart. This horizontal bar chart plots resources against elapsed time. Figure 5.3 shows an example of Gantt charts for project phases. These charts clearly communicate how many people will be involved in each phase of a project, the project components that are underway at any point in time, and even how much effort is required of any given project staff member.

The shaded areas in these charts represent time "cushions." These cushions are the time between the expected date of completion of a project component and the time when it is crucial for the component to be done for use in a later stage of the project. For example, consider the development of an imaging center. The first step is to develop a petition to the state for authorization. If the deadline for this is six months away, and you estimate that it will take only three months to complete the petition, then there is a cushion of three months, during which revisions can be made or project staff can be assigned other responsibilities.

A useful tool for communicating a project's costs and resource allocation is to develop a project control matrix. This matrix will clearly lay out cost and resource use by major category and plot them by project phase from the project activity chart. Figure 5.4 gives an example of this matrix, which allows each manager involved in the project to plan accurately how much money will be spent and how much payroll will be allocated to the project in each activity. After a quick look at the PAM, the manager also knows when in the fiscal cycle to budget for those costs.

Help with Project Planning. The planning of project details can be time consuming. This process becomes more demanding when one considers the dynamic nature of the health care provider. In many health care projects, plans must frequently be revised to accommodate shortages in available personnel, changes in state regulations, or the sometimes volatile staffing patterns in administrative suites. When these and myriad other realities of health care occur, the project manager is responsible for assessing their impact on the project, modifying

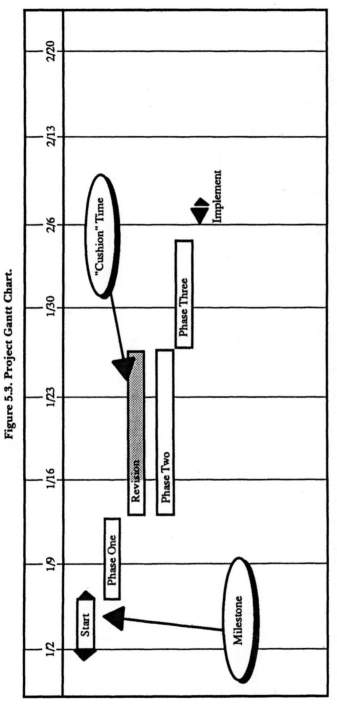

Figure 5.3. Project Gantt Chart.

Figure 5.4. Project Control Matrix.

Task Name	Days	Fixed Cost	Payroll	Resource 1	Resource 2	Resource 3	Resource 4
Start	2	5000	3150	Manager	Person 1	Person 2	Person 3
Phase One	5	7500	2750	Person 1	Person 3		
Revision	3	10000	750	Person 2			
Phase Two	10	20000	5750	Person 4	Person 2		
Phase Three	7	15000	7000	Person 1	Person 3	Manager	
Implement	1	2500	1250	Manager	Person 1	Person 2	Person 3

plans to compensate, and quickly communicating these revisions to all project and client personnel.

At such times the microcomputer becomes an invaluable management tool. Using project management software packages, the manager can quickly revise the plan and communicate it to all concerned parties. These software programs vary from product to product, but, in general, they share several capabilities: charting features; the ability to track event calendars, individual project staff time, and costs by project phase and by project staff; and the ability to automatically update all plans affected by the change in a single element, such as the number of staff available to work on one phase of the project. In addition, certain programs also enable the manager to compare planned events with actual project performance. As such, these tools are useful to assess and provide feedback on potential trouble spots in a project.

The project's complexity and the manager's facility with microcomputers will determine the choice of project management software. A manager with a large project who is relatively facile with computers might elect to use Project Manager's Workbench, which is very detailed in its treatment of the planning process and is well suited for large projects. The manager who is unfamiliar with DOS or who has a small- to medium-sized project might prefer a Macintosh-compatible system, such as MacProject. This package is among the easiest to use and provides excellent charting capabilities.

Pulling the Plan Together: The Work Plan. Once a project manager has determined who will be doing what to get a project completed, developing a work plan will help him to track progress compared to the original plan, understand and correct the causes of any delays, and effectively communicate with project staff and clients. The master work plan for the project is a matrix listing the steps in the project vertically along the left and, for each step, the individual responsible for its completion, the expected date of completion, the current date, and the current status of the step. At this level, the work plan allows the project manager to quickly determine where the project is, where management attention is needed, and who is working in each step. The work plan can and should be carried to the level of individual staff person, listing in chronological order the work and delivery date expectations for each person in the project.

Project Communication

If properly managed, project communication can be the greatest asset the manager has in coming through on time and within budget for a client. If not properly managed, however, communication will surely be the most frequent cause of project delays. Much of the planning process just presented is an iterative process of communication between the project manager and the administrator and between the project manager and the project team. There are typically five levels of communication to manage on a health care project:

- Between project manager and client (generally administration)
- Between project manager and staff manager
- Between project manager and project staff
- Between staff manager and staff (nonproject communication)
- Between project team and the institution

With all of these areas, the need for communication is constant, but most intense at the beginning and end phases of the project.

Rather than present traditional models of communication, I will provide a list of six practical suggestions for improving communication during a project.

1. Provide written follow-up on *all* communications with the client and with staff managers, particularly in the planning stages of the project. This may seem tedious, but reiteration of your understanding of scheduling and objectives can only help ensure that a project is proceeding as planned.
2. Conduct regularly scheduled project management meetings in which all staff managers and the project manager

participate. These meetings should be followed with written minutes distributed to all involved managers.

3. Schedule informal meetings with individual staff managers to discuss the impact of the project on their areas, the needs of their staff who are or will be assigned to the project, and any other issues important to each staff manager. Written follow-up for these meetings is not usually required unless the meeting results in a plan for action.

4. Arrange formal staff meetings at which the project manager and the entire project staff discuss their progress, any open issues, and ideas for their resolution. Do not have staff managers regularly participate in these staff meetings.

5. Conduct "management by walking around" tours of the project's work areas daily to discuss the project with individual staff members. This is an effective way to observe work quality, help resolve problems, and provide project staff with an opportunity to discuss individual problems they may not care to present at an all-staff meeting.

6. Control communication between the project team and the organization. This is critical in long projects and important on all projects. Most health care organizations are politically charged places, with everyone from staff physicians and various departments to the competitor down the street trying to find out "what those guys are *really* up to." Plan regularly scheduled communications with the organization as a whole and monthly updates for both the management staff and the medical staff of the hospital. Use the expertise of the provider's public relations department to plan and develop communications for the organization and, if appropriate, for the community's press. This will help ensure that the information you are providing will not be misunderstood and that it is received most favorably for the purposes of the project. If appropriate, monitor and limit all project team communication about project specifics to areas that are uncontroversial or already public knowledge.

This final item is not anywhere near as paranoiac as it sounds. Within one week prior to writing this chapter, I received two phone calls about this issue. One was from the vice president of planning and marketing at "Spys Are Us" Medical Center, and one was from a physician at a second hospital in the community. Both callers were trying to pump me for information about the activities of a project consultant at the physician's hospital. One of the callers suggested that I could help him discover (and find out for myself too) what the hospital was doing with the consultant and why. One caller was looking for competitive information, but the other may have been trying to learn how he would be affected by the project. If the effect would not be beneficial in his eyes, he may try to thwart the project and its manager.

Surveying Project Progress

Surveying a project is the process of monitoring four areas of project performance: actual versus planned production of objectives, actual versus planned cost of the project, project team satisfaction, and client/organizational satisfaction (including physicians, managers, employees, and the community). The manager surveying the actual versus planned production of objectives asks herself the following questions: "How far have we come, and how far do we have to go?" "How many steps have we completed?" and of great importance "Are we on time?" To make this determination, the project manager can generally rely upon well-maintained project work plans, which are updated regularly by staff.

Actual versus planned project expenditures can be determined from accounting reports for project activities. In organizations where accounting support cannot track and report specific project costs, the project manager must maintain detailed records of project costs in at least three areas: personnel time costs (including benefits) for all internal staff assigned to the project, consultant time and related costs, and equipment and capital costs. Many treatments of project management advocate a more rigorous accounting structure for managers of projects. Over half of the health care provider organizations in the nation are under 150 beds in size, however, and managers in these organizations are already wearing several hats. I see no need to make the health care manager a space-age accountant as well.

Project team satisfaction is one of the most delicately balanced facets of a project. Without a favorable report here, no manager will ever complete even the simplest project on time or to acceptable levels of quality. To assess team satisfaction, the project manager must rely upon reports by staff managers, direct communication with staff, and observations while wandering around project work areas. How do observations indicate staff satisfaction? Managers who make these observations and translations are effective with their staff. Those who do not are not. Key indicators of staff satisfaction include changes in staff promptness: Do typically reliable performers suddenly begin showing up late and leaving early? Topics of conversation and the pace of work are other indicators. Does conversation tend toward complaint and derisiveness? Is an area or part of the project team slow in accomplishing objectives without identifiable cause?

Entire texts have been written about staff job satisfaction and client satisfaction, for project managers and staff managers alike. An excellent discussion of project team and client satisfaction is provided by Hastings and others in *The Superteam Solution: Successful Teamworking in Organisations* (1986). *Practical Project Management* by Page-Jones (1985) presents strategies for managing staff satisfaction and staff development on a project team.

Coaching as a managerial tool has been written about in both conceptual articles in management periodicals and procedural guides for managerial skill building. Rather than belabor this important but much discussed skill, I refer the reader to two of the best treatments of the issue I have seen published. The first of these is *Performance Management: Improving Quality and Productivity through Positive Reinforcement* by Daniels and Rosen (1984). This text addresses the global issue of performance management and details the most crucial aspects of coaching from that perspective. The second text is *Supervisory Management for Healthcare Institutions* by Haimann (1973). This book is recommended because it presents the issue of managerial coaching from the perspective of differences in managerial styles and is directed to a health care audience.

Revising the Project

Change is the only constant in health care, and the project manager's challenge is to revise project activities' plans to accommodate that change. There are three general areas in which the manager may elect to revise a project, depending upon its progress. These areas are the scope of the project, the resources needed to complete the project, and the timing of activities. Feedback from clients, managers, and staff of a project, along with personal observations and management data, generally provide guidance as to what needs revision and how it might be revised. What I will focus on here is a short discussion of the nature and implications of revisions in each of these three areas.

Project scope should be revised, if at all, only in the earliest stages of the project. Generally, a manager may begin to have doubts about the feasibility of a project's scope as soon as she hears the client's request. This feeling often is not specific, but is founded in the manager's intimate understanding of the organizational dynamics and work patterns of the provider. It is generally best to validate these concerns through initial project planning before expressing a belief that revision of scope is necessary. Clients in general and physicians and administrators in particular will need specific evidence before they consider changing the scope of a project.

Resources needed to complete a project will undoubtedly need revising on at least a short-term level and occasionally on a long-term level as well. Short-term modifications to resource needs often occur in the area of staffing expertise required to handle a project phase in the allocated time line or as a result of unforeseen complications. These are best handled with individual staff managers. If staff are unavailable from internal sources, the manager may be forced to choose between revising project time lines, if there is any "play" in those schedules, and bringing in staff from outside the organization on temporary basis. The latter choice quickly translates into a cost issue and one of orienting consultants to the project and the organization.

Revising the timing of some or all project activities is often necessary because of unforeseen events within the team or changes in the environment outside of the project team. An example of timing changes caused by internal forces is the delay in a start-up of a project phase because of slower than expected progress by other staff working on a preceding component. Timing changes imposed on projects from the outside include slowed construction of a new clinic due to bad weather or labor problems and changes in legal requirements such as the certificate of need process in a particular state. In general, timing and resource revisions are interdependent; a change in one will require a change in the other. When timing revisions will delay a project milestone, the manager will need to negotiate alternatives to solving the problem with administrative officers, clients, or both.

Summary

The successful management of projects embodies the definition of a competent health care manager. While many managers may not have considered themselves project managers, every time they managed the care of a single patient, they in essence managed a project. The concepts and skills discussed in this chapter serve to expand the manager's role from patient-specific projects to efforts complicated by a greater number of external variables requiring guidance, control, and leadership. These projects demand careful planning and influencing of activities, people, resources, and communication in many technically different, highly autonomous areas within the health care delivery system.

To succeed in this environment, the health care manager must carefully develop an organizational structure and detailed work plan to support the project team's work. The project manager must carefully survey the project's development and progress and revise plans and activities as needed until the project succeeds. Finally, the manager must then ensure effective communication with the project's clients in the organization, administrative officers, the project team, and the organization as a whole. These issues, touched upon briefly here, are also discussed in greater detail in Chapters Three and Six.

6

❧

Building Teams:
The New Management Imperative

In Chapter Five, which addressed issues affecting the success of a project, I cited the project staff and the project team as key agents in such success. A project team is a unique instance of a team in the health care provider, but it is only one of many forms a team will take. Today's manager is a part of at least three ongoing teams at all times in addition to any special project teams he may lead or be a part of. These three ongoing teams include the department team, which the manager leads, the management team, composed of all department managers and staff administrative personnel, and the interdisciplinary patient care team. The manager's role in this last team is that of a staff manager, providing technical experts from department staff to various patient care areas.

With different roles in several teams, the manager needs to understand team dynamics and how teams are evaluated in a provider organization. This chapter does not attempt to present a comprehensive treatment of team management. Rather, the focus is specifically on the most timely and challenging issues affecting team performance in health care. I deal here with the management of ongoing teams in the provider organization, but many of the concepts and issues addressed for these teams also affect project teams.

What Is a Team?

What makes a team different from any other group of people? How can you tell a strong team from an ineffective one? The phrase "the health care team" has become almost a cliché. A true health care team is composed of not just physicians in a medical team, or nurses in a nursing team, or dieticians and staff in a dietary team. When we think about the teams we work with in hospitals, often our focus is on people of similar skills and interests—the people in our department. But the health care team is composed of a nurse, *and* a physician, *and* a dietician, *and* the marketing expert, *and* anyone else with special talents to complement, rather than duplicate, other team members. The purpose of the health care team is to focus the energies of the different talents needed to provide the best possible health care. A team with such diverse members presents many challenges to the health care manager who wants to ensure compassionately delivered, demographically specific services.

A team is defined as a group of people of divergent talents who must accomplish a common goal that cannot be achieved without cooperative, interdependent behavior. There are two primary types of teams to be managed: the department and the health care team. The department team contains the staff of specialists in any given area. Whether that area is facilities support or anesthesia is irrelevant. The department team's goal is prompt, client-centered special services of top quality. The health care team, composed of all of the players necessary to provide health care to the community, is much more dynamic and diverse than the department team. The precise talents represented on the health care team will change, depending upon the project or service undertaken. For example, the patient care health care team includes a physician, at least one nurse, usually other allied health professionals, dietary support staff, and the facilities and house-keeping personnel who will maintain the patient's physical environment. All of these talents must work side by side (literally at times) in an interdependent fashion to provide top-quality patient care. At another level, that of service planning, the team changes and includes physicians,

administrative executives, marketing professionals, and perhaps community and patient advocates. The goal of the health
care team is to provide for the community (whether that community is a single patient or an entire town) health care that is
medically flawless and emotionally supportive.

How Are Teams Evaluated?

Teams are evaluated at several levels, and to manage a
team, one must be aware of and apply criteria from all of these
levels. The three most important levels of evaluation of team
effectiveness are client, organizational, and internal team
evaluations.

Who are clients and how do they evaluate a health care
team? Clients are the patient, the family of the patient, and other
organizational staff who will be around to observe at least the
effects of the services rendered, if not the actual services. Clients'
observations and evaluations of the quality of a department
team will be as varied as the clients themselves. But at many levels
and many times each day, the department team is being evaluated. Whether the criterion for evaluation is a sticky floor beside
a patient's bed or a brusque, uncommunicative physician, the
quality of health care teams is constantly assessed.

Even though some of the criteria may seem to have little to
do with the quality of the health care team, they are the basis for
the client passing final judgment on the team. The patient and
family hold special importance among team clients; they are
"preferred customers" of sorts. The patient's evaluation of health
care is very different from that of anyone who works in a hospital. The patient is unaware of the technical issues of medical
quality. In the absence of information about this, the patient and
family evaluate the quality of their medical care by criteria with
which they are familiar. Whether or not these criteria are relevant to actual team performance in a medical sense, judgment is
passed. The patient is the ghostwriter of the manager's paycheck,
and so, for very selfish reasons, the manager has a vested interest
in understanding how this client evaluates health care.

In one survey of the lay public, Lombardi (1984) determined the most important criteria used by patients and their families when evaluating health care teams. Regardless of geographic location, the top four ways people determine whether they have received high quality medical care are:

- Compassion shown by staff
- Time spent with patient
- Ready answers to questions
- Length of time spent waiting to be served

In another survey of over 1,000 people conducted in 1985, the key determinants of patient satisfaction with health care services were staff communication skills and the skill of *individual* staff members, as perceived by patients and families. Overall care quality as an independent criterion was a distant third in importance. The consistent feature in all patient definitions of quality care is the importance of customer satisfaction.

What are the implications for the health care manager? In addition to using budget performance, Joint Committee for the Accreditation of Healthcare Organizations compliance, morbidity and mortality statistics, and quality assurance assessments of team performance, he had better assess the quality of team performance as defined by the patient. This may have been a "nice" thing to do ten years ago, and a "revolutionary" concept in the industry eight years ago, but today it is a basic requirement of health care team assessment—and will be in the future. Indeed, this customer service assessment model should be expanded to include all people and organizations served by the manager's department.

The first step in evaluating the customer service performance is to identify the customers served by a team. This list should include both internal and external customers. Internal customers are any other employee or attending physician in an institution. For example, internal customers of a medical laboratory include physicians, nurses, and therapists who rely upon the laboratory for information about their patients. Patients and their families are external clients.

In addition to identifying who the customers of a depart-

Exhibit 6.1. Customer Service Quality Assessment Instrument.

Department Team Customer Service

Internal Customer Groups	Success Factors for Group	Current Satisfaction				
		1 Low	2	3	4	5 High
1. _____	_____					
	_____					
	_____					
2. _____	_____					
	_____					
	_____					
3. _____	_____					
	_____					
	_____					

External Customer Groups	Success Factors for Group	Current Satisfaction				
		1 Low	2	3	4	5 High
1. _____	_____					
	_____					
	_____					
2. _____	_____					
	_____					
	_____					
3. _____	_____					
	_____					
	_____					

ment team are, it is also important to identify the critical indica-tors of team performance from the perspective of each cus-tomer and their current perceptions. The tool in Exhibit 6.1 can be used to accomplish this.

Besides identifying a team's customers, the manager must determine how those customers evaluate the service provided by the department (or other) team. This can be done from two perspectives: how the manager and the team *think* the customer group will evaluate team performance and how that group actually assesses the team. While the latter is more precise, conducting both evaluations can provide important information for the manager, and the difference between team perceptions and reality is a useful tool to focus the team's energy on developing their customer service skills.

The manager may also wish to help her team focus on customer support by having each team member assess his or her individual mind-set toward customer service. This assessment is enlightening in many industries where customer service is a mainstay of business growth, but in health care, many teams find the prospect of evaluating their "readiness to serve customers" as opposed to "care for patients" a revolutionary idea. Participating in this revolution, however, often helps individuals and entire teams rethink their approach to health care, allowing them to embrace the notion of *serving* clients who are patients, physicians, and others, rather than paternalistically *caring* for the ill. Exhibit 6.2 shows one tool for evaluating readiness to serve clients. This simple questionnaire, which should take no more than ten minutes to complete, can be helpful in beginning a process in which staff can reflect on service issues and start self-assessment. The survey is designed for self-assessment by staff only.

The Relationship Between Team Effectiveness and Customer Service

What does a manager do if her team's track record at customer service is not up to speed? There are generally three possible interpretations of low customer service performance by a team. One is unclear or constantly changing expectations by the manager for customer service performance. Until recently, most health care personnel never thought twice about customer service. Why should they? They did not work with customers—they worked with doctors and patients. Many customer service deficits in health care do not indicate team dysfunction at all. They can be the result of a lack of staff under-

Exhibit 6.2. Evaluating Customer Service Readiness in Team Members.

Self-Assessment: My Internal Mind-Set to Support Service

Circle the extent you agree or disagree with each statement.

	Disagree			Agree	
1. There is nothing demeaning about assisting or serving others.	1	2	3	4	5
2. I can be cheerful and positive to everyone regardless of age, appearance, race, gender, and class.	1	2	3	4	5
3. On bad days when nothing goes right, I can still find ways to be positive.	1	2	3	4	5
4. The higher the quality of service I provide while I'm at work the better I feel.	1	2	3	4	5
5. I am enthusiastic about my job.	1	2	3	4	5
6. Encountering difficult "people" situations from time to time will not cause me to be negative.	1	2	3	4	5
7. The idea of being a professional at customer service is motivating to me.	1	2	3	4	5
8. Performing a "people-oriented" job is both challenging and fun.	1	2	3	4	5
9. I feel great pleasure and pride when people compliment me or my organization for superior service.	1	2	3	4	5
10. Doing well in all aspects of my job is important to me.	1	2	3	4	5

TOTAL SCORE __ __ __ __ __

Total

Add the columns down, and then add
these totals for a Total Score.

Scoring:
If you scored above 40, you currently have personal resources that should
help you to be effective and able to cope with the stress of customer
service work.

If you scored between 25 and 40, you may be experiencing significant
stress in the delivery of customer service on a daily basis.

A rating below 25 may indicate that the stress caused by direct customer
service work could reduce your effectiveness on the job.

Source: Adapted from Martin (1987).

standing of expectations about customer service performance. Before a manager jumps directly from the signs of deficiencies to prescribing training or team-building interventions for staff, she should first make certain that she has clearly explained the team's roles and responsibilities in the area of customer service. It is even more effective for the manager and her team to cooperatively establish standards for customer service quality. A second interpretation of poor service is a lack of training in the behavioral skills of customer service. Most health care staff are very adept at highly technical and demanding disciplines. They are adept because they have studied and practiced these skills until they are nearly automatic. Few people in health care have had the luxury of training for and practice at managing irate customers or any of the other skills associated with customer service. A third possibility: If skills are in place, and staff members clearly understand performance expectations, then poor performance in this area by a team may indicate a need for team development. Team development will help to produce a cohesive group of people who focus on common goals and support each other in achieving those goals. If skills and knowledge are in place and the goals of customer service are not being met, then it is time to examine the possible causes and rectify them.

Evaluating an Effective Health Care Team

How does one tell whether a team is really a team or simply a group of people with a profession or employer in common? A real team is an action-oriented, mutually supportive group willing to go the extra mile to meet priority goals. Now a manager cannot very well ask his staff if they are dynamic and willing to go the extra mile, because team support is to organizational culture what patriotism is to the Marine Corps. The manager would undoubtedly get a resounding cry of "yes, sir!" until he left the room. The health and well-being of a team can be diagnosed by studying the team's vital signs even as a person's health can be crudely gauged using more traditional vital signs. The two types of team vital signs, described by MacGregor

(1967), that a manager should monitor are personal characteristics and group traits.

The personal characteristics present in every member of
an effective health care team involve understanding, support,
trust, and openness. Mutual understanding and active support
of the team's primary goal is especially important for clinical
teams because while there are stable long-term team goals, the
short-term goals of the team can change minute by minute.
Everyone working in the emergency room must have the same
understanding of which case needs attention first and what the
most urgent care needs are for any given patient. Complete trust
in all other team members can be seen in activities unrelated to
teamwork such as in social situations. This trust is often evident
in effective critical care teams, but is equally important on
planning and administrative teams, whose members must trust
that the others are going to provide the support that they will
need to be successful. Members of an effective team also communicate freely about goal-related issues, even unpleasant issues.
This openness is not the same as a willingness to criticize team
members. Communication in an effective team is based on
respect and trust that even criticism is offered for the good of the
project and the team member. Another sign of an effective team
is willingness to support the activities and resolve problems of
other team members. There is no need to elaborate on ways a
manager can determine the willingness of team members to go
the extra mile. All that is needed is a staffing shortage caused by
a flu epidemic or a heavy patient load in the unit.

Group traits that are vital to effective team functioning
are also well documented. These include its skills, problem-
solving abilities, and leadership. Team members as a group
possess the wide variety of skills necessary to accomplish the
team's goal. This does not mean that team members have the
same skills or that each member has a talent unique to himself,
although either of these structures might work. Chapter Seven,
dealing with subordinate training and development, contains a
process and tools for determining department competency
needs that a manager can easily use when planning team composition. An effective team can identify the causes and creatively

resolve the differences that arise among its members, rather than fail to address differences or openly criticize each other. This characteristic relies heavily upon two individual characteristics: open communication and trust in each team member. In effective teams, a clearly defined leader is responsible for maintaining the traits of an effective team as the group's norm and making decisions about the team's direction. This definition of leadership says nothing about the managerial functions necessary for successful health care management. The team's leader may influence the management of a department and does not necessarily have to be the manager.

Decision Making for Effective Teamwork

Although the team leader is ultimately responsible for all team decisions, a wise team leader uses her team selectively to achieve time-efficient, intelligent decisions and maintain team cohesiveness. Decision-making styles occur along a continuum, as Figure 6.1 shows. Each style on the continuum is valid and can be used effectively in different environments. Each also has predictable characteristic patterns regarding who makes decisions in a department and how those decisions are communicated to team members. While comparing the examples in Figure 6.1, one should also consider the fact that in some organizations the preferred decision-making style is to not make decisions at all. In this style a team leader simply avoids making and implementing a decision until the environment makes it for him.

Every leader has a preferred style of decision making and team leadership that is used routinely in day-to-day activities. A preferred decision-making style does not mean that a person is wed exclusively to that style and cannot use another decision-making process. To be an effective health care team leader, the manager must understand what her preferred style of making decisions is and when to use it or another style of decision making.

Team members as individuals and as a group have very strong reactions to leadership decision-making practices. Health

Decision-Making Style	Extreme autocratic	Consultative	Consensus	No one decides
Decision Maker	Team leader	Team leader	Team group	N/A
Team Communication	Not informed of leader's decisions	Consulted during decision-making process	Consulted during process, recommends decision as a group.	N/A

care teams are usually composed of extremely bright, self-possessed professionals who need input into significant decisions that will affect the team's mission. Failure to effectively involve team members in making decisions is one of the greatest threats to effective team functioning in health care, particularly when the team has one or more physicians.

On the continuum of decision-making styles, from autocratic to laissez-faire, the styles most effective in health care teams depend upon the nature of the task the team is facing. Using the appropriate decision-making style is critically important to health care team leadership. Three general guidelines for effective decision making by the type of decisions to be made are listed below.

When does a team leader seek group consensus before reaching a decision, and when does the leader retain the prerogative of position and make decisions alone? Burke (1982) suggested three conditions under which an effective team leader will seek the consensus of team members before reaching a decision:

1. When he does not know which group member has the most expertise in an area.
2. When implementing the decision will require time and support from several team members.
3. When a decision must be made rapidly, and there is little or no time to gather hard data. In this situation, the judgments and opinions of team members can serve as a starting point from which to reach consensus with greater perspective and wisdom than that of the leader alone.

These three guidelines are sound and strongly recommended for managing team decision making. One unique aspect of health care teams and their decision making that merits further elaboration is the involvement of allied health professionals and, more significantly, physicians.

Physicians and Allied Health Professionals: Unique Team-Building Considerations

By the nature of their work and training, health professionals must regularly make important decisions autonomously. Although there are guidelines for making these decisions, data must be collected, analyzed, and interpreted on a case-by-case basis by the individual care giver. This autonomy is guarded vociferously. Health care professionals cannot work effectively in a trusting team if they fear even a temporary loss of this decision-making autonomy. But how does one manage a team of these professionals and allow each of them autonomy over decision making?

While there is no one correct approach to this challenge, several guidelines are very effective if modified by the team leader to accommodate his personal decision-making style, the needs of the project, and the individual needs of team members. First, establish clear guidelines regarding individual decision-making protocol and communication of decisions to all team members. While the leader must make decisions about the overall direction of team activities, these decisions need only focus on four areas of team performance: team organization and communication protocol, work schedules for team members' objectives, allocation of resources for work, and communications with nonteam members about team activities. In general, the team leader will move the team along to success if he manages the administrative functions of team leadership in an autocratic fashion, seeking input as appropriate but reserving the decisions to himself.

Decisions about how a task or objective should be accomplished are another matter entirely. These decisions, regarding how team members should accomplish tasks and objectives, are often best made by the individual team members. This will allow the team members to determine their own priorities and how they do their job. If possible, define the roles of physicians on the team to allow them maximum opportunity to interpret information, react to developments, and recommend alternatives. Let them use the diagnostic and prescriptive strengths they apply in their medical practices on a day-to-day basis.

If at all feasible, share team leadership with all team members by establishing a structure that rotates leadership according to expertise. For example, when addressing the nursing issues, a nurse on the team would lead team planning and discussion. When dealing with the marketing of medical services, the team member from marketing would lead activities. In this structure, the team leader would guide the process of team activities and meetings, rather than make decisions in technical areas in which she is not an expert.

Building Team Performance

How one builds an effective team depends on the individuals involved and the issues that the team faces. Guidelines for team building and maintenance are provided here and described according to the problems in the team's performance that will indicate a need for team building.

The number and variety of problems that can develop in a team are endless. I will focus on four of the most frequently occurring problems a team may encounter and provide specific recommendations for team development interventions for each.

General development guidelines, which apply to all team building issues, are summed up in three steps:

1. Identify the team performance issue. While the team leader may have a very good idea of what the problem is and what the most effective corrective measures would be, she must help all team members recognize that a problem exists and that they must explore solution alternatives together. When a team performance issue develops, the team leader should have already established group norms that value total team ownership of any individual team member's problems—if it's his problem, it's my problem.
2. Develop a consensus of the causes of the performance issue and alternatives for its solution. The greatest danger to the team at this point, particularly a recently established team,

is finger pointing in which team members blame each other for performance problems. The goal of the team leader is to force the team to focus on problems as events and not people. This can be facilitated by having all team members ask themselves several key questions: What events occurred that resulted in this issue? What could I have done to help avoid any of those events? What could any of my team members have done to help avoid those events? What other factors are affecting this situation, and how can we as a team influence them?

3. Develop a plan to remove any barriers to team performance using the issues identified by the team. This is not a consensus operation in project teams, but at the team leader's discretion, may be a shared team responsibility.

Problem: Cannot Get Past First Base (or Second, or Third)

The problem of slowed progress is frustrating at any point in a project, but it can be totally demoralizing to team members in the start-up phase. Although most recommendations for team leadership advocate sharing decision making and rotating leadership by team members' expertise, if a problem with progress develops, the team leader must quickly focus the team's energy and prioritize its objectives.

The primary indications of a team suffering from a lack of progress are conflicting priorities among team members, frequently "refined" objectives and goals, and false starts. A common indicator of the latter is the team that meets several times to address similar agenda items. The team leader's responsibility to a team that cannot get past first base is to be an aggressive process facilitator while protecting the team from organizational pressures and each other. Specific steps to resolution include gate-keeping, or controlling the access of outsiders to the team. This includes administrative officers and medical staff especially, who frequently have a high need for information and a high need to influence the direction or activities of the team. Another step is to facilitate communication between team members and, if necessary, improve the flow of information to the team. Frequently, one of the causes of the delayed starts and team floundering is an inability of team members to get commitment needed for them to proceed. This can range from a physician not certain about a diagnosis to a CEO who is supporting a project only because she is pressured by influential physicians.

Problem: Turf Wars

Turf wars are loud, ugly, and painful to team members in addition to being destructive to team performance. The eruption of conflict or more subtle hindrance of progress by one or more groups, turf wars are particularly delicate situations for the team leader to manage. Unfortunately, health care delivery systems are especially vulnerable to the occasional outbreak of turf wars, largely because of a heavy reliance on different professionals who are at once very autonomous and clear about their professional identity and coincidentally have overlapping areas of expertise. The question at hand in most health care turf wars is stated as "Who is more qualified and therefore should be responsible to do this?" The message often intentionally implied in this statement is "*I* am more qualified than you are to manage this highly responsible task." To a health care professional who defines herself by her work expertise, "them's fightin' words."

Turf wars can erupt within the team between members, between the team and others in the organization who are not part of the team, and — most dangerously to team functioning — between one team member or group and another team faction siding with an external group. Signs and symptoms of a turf war include derisive statements and behavior or statements that blow things out of proportion when describing problems involving others. Withholding or manipulating needed information until it is not useful and failing to respond to requests for support ("If you're so good, what do you need me for?") are other signs of a turf war. Some conflicts produce "prophets of doom," always predicting (hoping for) total, demoralizing failure with serious repercussions to the organization ("Then they'll be sorry!"). The team leader's role in a turf war, like the police in a riot, is first to restore peace and then to pick up the pieces. It is much wiser, however, for the health care leader to take steps to avoid the development of turf wars, at least those internal to the team.

Assuming the absence of any preexisting political agendas, turf wars erupt generally because involved parties are insecure in their own minds about their value to the team's talent pool, unable to see the value of members with different professional backgrounds but who have talents that overlap theirs, or unable to understand or appreciate the personal strengths of the individuals who serve as their adversaries. As noted earlier, project teams come together precisely because of the members' different talents. The same is true to varying degrees in permanent teams. Even when the different members of a permanent team have similar functions, each person brings to that function unique assets and liabilities that can complement the liabilities and assets of other team members.

To take advantage of these complementary strengths and weaknesses, however, the team leader and all team members must understand them and how they are best used. For example, a team member who relies on hard fact and deductive logic might be an excellent diagnostician. These talents do not always go hand in hand with interpersonal sensitivity and diplomacy. But with both talents in different members of a team, the team can be effective in recommending treatment for patients and in diplomatically presenting these recommendations to attending physicians. They can be effective, however, only when both team members understand the individual strengths and weaknesses of each other and how they can work together.

To help team members understand the unique personal strengths and liabilities they each bring to the team, the manager may consider using a Myers-Briggs Type Indicator (MBTI). The MBTI is a profiling system that accurately measures individual personality types by four criteria:

- How an individual gathers information
- Where an individual focuses attention in problem solving and related activities

- How an individual typically makes decisions
- The way a person interacts with others

In the Myers-Briggs Type Indicator system, every person's personality type is expressed as a function of the four traits identified above. Each of these traits, or types, is a continuum between two extremes, as follows:

I (Introvert) through E (Extrovert)
S (Sensing) through N (Intuitive)
T (Thinking) through F (Feeling)
J (Judging) through P (Perceiving)

Each person's profile is expressed by some combination of these four types. For example, one person's type profile might be ENTJ, using the symbols above, while another might be ISFP. Each combination of personality-type characteristics carries with it predictable assets for team performance, which can be balanced by other types to create a team tailored to the challenge facing the manager.

The MBTI, when properly administered in a team development situation, allows team members to discover the different personality characteristics they and their teammates bring to the team. The MBTI clearly describes both assets and liabilities. This allows the team to explore the merits of a mix of different types of people in a team and the value of each member. Used proactively, it also allows a manager to select team members who bring complementary individual strengths to the overall team function. Table 6.1 provides a general description of the variety of MBTI types and the assets each type brings to a team. Keep in mind that these descriptions are generalizations of the MBTI and that the instrument measures much more precisely the personal attributes of team members than can be reflected here.

A practical alternative to avoiding turf wars on a team is to build in each team member an appreciation for the technical skills of all team members. This can be accomplished by rotating team members through daily work with each of their teammates as observers. The orientation to teammates' work would provide

Table 6.1. Myers-Briggs Type Characteristics in Summary.

Contribution Made by Each Myers-Briggs Type Preference

Sensing Types		*Intuitive Types*	
Combined with Thinking	*Combined with Feeling*	*Combined with Feeling*	*Combined with Thinking*
ISTJ I Depth of concentration S Reliance on facts T Logic and analysis J Organization	**ISFJ** I Depth of concentration S Reliance on facts F Warmth and sympathy J Organization	**INFJ** I Depth of concentration N Grasp of possibilities F Warmth and sympathy J Organization	**INTJ** I Depth of concentration N Grasp of possibilities T Logic and analysis J Organization
ISTP I Depth of concentration S Reliance on facts T Logic and analysis P Adaptability	**ISFP** I Depth of concentration S Reliance on facts F Warmth and sympathy P Adaptability	**INFP** I Depth of concentration N Grasp of possibilities F Warmth and sympathy P Adaptability	**INTP** I Depth of concentration N Grasp of possibilities T Logic and analysis P Adaptability
ESTP E Breadth of interests S Reliance on facts T Logic and analysis P Adaptability	**ESFP** E Breadth of interests S Reliance on facts F Warmth and sympathy P Adaptability	**ENFP** E Breadth of interests N Grasp of possibilities F Warmth and sympathy P Adaptability	**ENTP** E Breadth of interests N Grasp of possibilities T Logic and analysis P Adaptability
ESTJ E Breadth of interests S Reliance on facts T Logic and analysis J Organization	**ESFJ** E Breadth of interests S Reliance on facts F Warmth and sympathy J Organization	**ENFJ** E Breadth of interests N Grasp of possibilities F Warmth and sympathy J Organization	**ENTJ** E Breadth of interests N Grasp of possibilities T Logic and analysis J Organization

Key to personality-type abbreviations: I = Introvert   E = Extrovert   T = Thinking   F = Feeling
S = Sensing   N = Intuitive   P = Perceiving   J = Judging

Source: Adapted from Briggs-Myers and McCauley, 1985.

an opportunity for each individual to demonstrate and explain the exact nature of her work. This immersion in the technical culture of different types of teammates helps break down the walls of professional parochialism that often fortify the camps of turf war combatants.

Regardless of how the team leader addresses the underlying causes of turf wars, when they develop, the job of the leader is clear:

1. Revise existing performance and behavior standards and norms for the team. Modify established standards or set new standards for the team.
2. Communicate these standards to the team and explain the need for them.
3. Allow the team an opportunity to develop an alternative to these standards that will work as well. The team leader should not assist the team with this task. The team leader can refuse the team's alternatives if he believes that they will not resolve the performance issues resulting from the turf war. This forces the team to either live under someone else's rule or its own and can often create cooperation among team members.
4. Encourage and support the team as a whole entity. Recognize the turf problems directly, but emphasize the "we" of a team.
5. Relieve the tension that will arise between parties involved in the conflict and that will affect other team members.

An excellent demonstration of a turf war is a case in which Our Lady of Lourdes Medical Center set out to establish a home health care service for their community. The service was to be comprehensive, providing parenteral nutrition, pulmonary care, chemotherapy, and physical therapy services to hospital patients after they left inpatient care status. The project team that planned the service was flawless in its delivery of a feasibility study, a preliminary site plan, and recommendations for service lines to be offered. The CEO of the medical center was very excited because the board wanted to proceed with the center's development immediately.

The CEO promoted the director of respiratory care to the position of assistant administrator, with responsibility for establishing and managing the center. This was done over the protests of one member of the hospital's executive staff. The director of nursing (DON) felt that because of the range of services and the need for nursing involvement in the delivery of home care services, the home health care center should be managed by someone with a broad base of experience in the various nursing competencies. The CEO's rationale for his decision was that his candidate of choice had a solid record for establishing new services in the hospital, had demonstrated a flair for marketing services to the medical staff and the community, and was one of the strongest managers of people on the administrative staff. He felt these skills were crucial because the staff of the home health care services would be a very mixed group and would be functioning with more autonomy and decision making than any of their peers working within the walls of the hospital. In addition, the director of respiratory care was a competent professional in his chosen technical discipline of cardiopulmonary therapy, which was where the greatest portion of home care services were rendered.

The problems that plagued the new assistant administrator as he began to plan staffing needs were myriad. A request for nursing policies and procedures from the oncology and enterostomal therapy units took eight weeks and four follow-up requests before it was met. Internal nursing candidates for staff at the home care center were nonexistent, despite the greater nursing freedom attached to the position and a much more stable work schedule. The new assistant administrator found the DON's calendar booked solid when he tried to set an appointment to discuss the center's needs and get planning input from her.

In this case, the DON was so upset that her advice was not heeded that she set up a system of informal communication and rumor in the nursing staff that paralyzed the new home care director in his efforts to plan nursing services for the center. A combination of the success of the home care administrator at obtaining cooperation and planning input from other depart- ments and subsequent intervention by the chief operating of- ficer resulted ultimately in a grudging level of cooperation from the DON, who would have been happier if the administrator had failed in his efforts to set up a home care service.

Problem: Burnout

Burnout, a term coined to describe the progressive decline of performance and commitment by typically stellar individuals and teams, is a problem plaguing many health care teams. While burnout affects all segments of society, it is much more frequent and destructive in environments of high stress and low recogni- tion, as frequently are found in health care.

Why do I describe health care as a low-recognition en- vironment? The performance standards for clinical providers are necessarily high. There is little margin for performance error when dealing with human life, and so each care giver is expected to perform all of his duties with flawless precision. It is often a manager's practice to acknowledge this performance as "acceptable" or as "meeting standards." No additional recogni- tion of the quality, care, and commitment is offered, because it is felt that none is warranted for performing to the same standards of excellence that all other team members are expected to meet.

Who is susceptible to burnout? What are the charac- teristics of the development of burnout in an individual or team, and what can the manager as a team leader do to prevent or correct the effects of burnout? Typically, burnout affects the most committed individuals in a team and the most dedicated teams in an organization. These teams and individuals are generally very task oriented and will sacrifice themselves and the norms of a group to achieve their goals. In fact, this extreme task orientation in an environment where management support and mutual effort by other team members is not visible is at the root of the problem of burnout in health care. Burnout can affect any team or any team member, but there is a typical pattern of burnout in an organization.

Burnout generally occurs most frequently to people in positions of high responsibility and accountability but little authority. This combination places a committed professional who is dedicated to success in work and improving the organiza- tion in a position where she has no authority to do so. When combined with an apparent lack of management support, the professional recognizes that successful change is unlikely and undesired by leaders. Nowhere is this more clearly seen than at the levels of allied health professional and staff administration in a health care provider. A quick review of various professional journals will indicate which professionals are at highest risk of burnout. These are the professions whose journals address the "management" of burnout by the affected individual and how to "avoid" burnout in their careers.

Appelbaum (1981) also suggested that clinical personnel in health care are generally more susceptible than are non- clinical personnel. Within the ranks of clinical personnel, those who routinely faced the management of critically ill patients were most likely to be affected by burnout. The reasons for this seem to be twofold. There is a paradox in the daily lives of clinical professionals that is difficult to resolve. The emphasis in daily work and in the social pecking order of clinical health care is on knowledge and ability to treat clinical disorders such as the "multiple trauma in bed 3" or the "collapsed lung in room 5." Clinical professionals are trained to believe that with enough medical knowledge and rapid intervention, they can restore a patient to health and well-being. Yet they fail at times. Some- times there is a reason that can be traced back to a care decision with which they did not agree. Sometimes there is no identifi- able cause for this failure. Both of these instances create feelings of impotence in the clinician.

These feelings of inadequacy and impotence are often compounded when clinicians, who again are trained and so- cialized to believe that medicine is a sort of twentieth-century magic that will restore their patients to well-being, find that they are totally unprepared to deal with painful problems faced by patients, particularly the chronically ill. These problems are of emotional dependency and a need for compassionate understanding. Clinicians may recognize a patient's need for this support, but often find it very difficult to change their approach from treating a disease to interacting with a human being in pain. Attempts to do this put the clinician in a position where she must not only recognize that she cannot remove the patient's emotional pain but also must face it and feel it to be of any comfort to the patient.

What are the characteristics of burnout, and how can burnout affect the team? Burnout can be suspected in teams or individuals where any of the following exist: slowing of momentum from an individual or team's typical pace, absence of additional effort in the face of new challenges, growing cynicism in individuals or the entire team, and expressed feelings of professional impotence. Other symptoms of burnout are the absence of management support or intervention to alleviate team problems or performance roadblocks and increasing isolation of team members from decision making and the communication of decisions affecting them.

Managing the problem of burnout is a complicated issue. The provider organization contains many of the factors that create situations where team members are chronically in positions of high responsibility and low authority. These factors are integral to the organizational culture and the nature of the work. Consistent, expedient patient care demands a single authority in the prescription of treatment. This paternalistic approach to medicine has become ingrained in the basic cultural structure of health care management. Although there are many creative and successful experiments to more effectively manage the delivery and management of health care, they are just that—experiments—and not yet inculcated into the mainstream of the very conservative culture of health care.

But there are steps a health care manager can take to deal with burnout in her staff. These steps include acknowledging the problem with the staff. Team members often will not want to acknowledge that there is anything out of the ordinary. The team leader must maintain an ongoing environment where expression of feelings is a safe and desirable thing for team members to do. The leader must stress that there is nothing inadequate in team members and that the system in which they are working does not deserve total rejection. The manager can protect her staff by being an aggressive gatekeeper. Very often, when progress slows, or work quality takes a temporary down-turn, political forces in an organization tend to start a witch-hunt, looking to condemn "the evil among us." The strong leader must serve as a barricade to keep these inquisitors from reaching her team. The only criticism to reach team members directly while a project is in process must come from the leader or peers within the team. The manager also should encourage communication between team members and investigate inci-dents cited by staff as significant to them in the development of burnout in their work. Finally, clinical team leaders can further support their teams in the avoidance of burnout through train-ing and management planning in the emotional and social implications of disease. Much clinical burnout can be addressed by teaching team members how to manage the "other" side of patient care — the emotional side. When team members under-stand the well-documented genesis of emotional and social dys-functions that occur in disease, they will be better prepared to help their patients with their stress and to avoid the threat of burnout.

Problem: Ivory Tower of Excellence

The Ivory Tower of Excellence is a seductive performance problem in American business, particularly health care. This is characterized by an highly uniform set of opinions among team members on nearly every issue relevant to their mission. The team typically enjoys a high morale and a cohesiveness that leads it to act defensively when faced with any expression of fact or opinion that does not conform to its views. The problem can affect a team or an entire organization; it leads to complacency and a smug feeling of invulnerability.

Because American cars had enjoyed a reputation for qual-ity for two decades, industry executives became complacent. They were so high in their Ivory Tower of Excellence that they failed to see a changing definition of excellence in their industry. In the 1950s and 1960s gasoline was inexpensive and few people were concerned about pollution. In this era "excellence" was defined as fast, heavy, and roomy. The advent of environ-mental awareness and the sharply rising cost of fuel, however, changed forever the definition of excellence for automotive consumers. The emerging definition, unheeded by American car makers, was small, fuel efficient, and safe. American car makers were not stupid; they simply did not face the facts in front of them because they were victims of this team perfor-mance problem. By the time American auto makers realized what had happened, retooled, and learned how to make fuel-efficient cars, they had lost nearly half of their customers.

Equivalents of this in health care include many institu-tional casualties where management teams in hospitals refused to take the threat of HMO development and private walk-in clinics seriously. After all, why would people even think about turning their backs on their community hospital for a rinky-dink little facility that could not offer half of the high-tech services available in the hospital? They never even considered that patients reacted to issues of cost and customer service. By refusing to recognize trends in patient traffic and underlying causes, many managers did not develop competitive strategies in time to stem the flow of patients from their facilities. This, combined with other industry pressures, put many hospitals in a position of playing catch-up, if not a position of bankruptcy, in the late 1970s and early 1980s.

Indicators that a manager's team may be suffering from this organizational narcissism include shared stereotypes of customers' values and competitors' capabilities that are not based on any contemporary empirical evidence and generally accepted rationalizations for team failures or lack of effective-ness. Another sign of the ivory-tower attitude is group rejection of individuals or information that presents reasonable but con-flicting conclusions, interpretations, or opinions about relevant issues. The team becomes a clique. This is a common develop-ment in internal teams of people in a service department. These teams view opinions of other professionals or departments as ignorant—unenlightened and undeserving serious consideration: "What do those nurses know about this anyway?" or "You know those marketing types. All they want us to do is smile at everyone—as if that's what patient care were all about" or "We can't do that. It would totally disrupt the way we do our work" are typical statements of the clique (even though the way we do our work might be better off if it were shaken up a bit occasionally).

The manager faced with the problem of an overly co-hesive team is a part of that team. In this position, it can be difficult to recognize the performance problem. Once it is rec-ognized, the leader must address the problem by forcing the team to consider outside information. It is important for the leader in this situation to refrain from leadership. To aggres-sively lead in adopting new information and perspectives might simply change the foundation of the ivory tower.

A team with the ivory-tower syndrome has unconsciously lost sight of its task. This team's mission has changed from accomplishing a goal to maintaining team integrity and social status quo. Their motto is "don't rock the boat." Because this team needs solid consensus on all issues to maintain co-hesiveness, members will be willing to change their opinions, if they are the opinions of a leader, and if they can change them quickly as a group. Therefore, the manager should actively seek unbiased external information sources that might conflict with the team's present opinion. If a team leader can bring in an outside speaker who will present objectively developed informa-tion conflicting with current team understanding of an issue, she can orchestrate the development of team consensus that is based upon an analysis of available data rather than a need to conform.

After sharing information from a source that the team generally accepts as credible, team members should not be allowed to discuss the issue together. Instead, they should each be instructed to develop their own interpretation of the infor-mation and recommendations based on that interpretation. Each of these recommendations should be prepared in writing and submitted within twenty-four hours.

The team leader can then review the recommendations and report to the team as a group. The team leader's report

should focus on the differences in each team member's recommendations and on oversights and possible errors in the logic of
individual team members. This can effectively force the team to
a consensus on the issues that is the result of intellectual examination, rather than peer conformity.

There are several strategies a manager can take to counter
the development of a team that becomes so cohesive as to be
insular. One strategy is to challenge the assumptions and conclusions of the team in each decision it makes. Demand empirical support for each conclusion it reaches, and present
conflicting evidence where available, asking team members to
resolve any conflicts presented. Another strategy is to assign
team members the tasks of critically evaluating the work of their
peers independently and of providing recommendations for
strengthening the results of that work. Make it clear to the
reviewers that their performance will be evaluated based on the
quantity and quality of their recommendations, while their
teammate's work will be evaluated on the overall quality of the
product after adopting appropriate recommendations for
improvement.

Throughout this process the manager must protect the
team from external criticism and undue influence from other
sources in the organization. Exposure to either legitimate or
inappropriate criticism from the outside will generally make the
ivory-tower team more difficult to manage. Such criticism easily
galvanizes a team as a means of protecting the individuals in the
group from the sting of the criticism.

Summary

Health care has professed a dedication to the "team approach" to healing for many years. Yet true teams in health
care—teams that are dynamic, cohesive, and goal oriented—are
a rare commodity. Among functional teams seen in many provider organizations, most are not oriented toward client service.
They are instead task oriented. Examples of these task-oriented
teams include those found in burn units, where teamwork is
focused on the treatment of a dysfunction, or in interdisciplin-

ary teams brought together for finite projects, such as installation of a new information system or establishing a new service line for the community.

The focus of this chapter has been on identifying priorities for building teams that will meet the emerging needs of the provider organization and its clients. These priorities include building a team that is oriented toward customer service, as well as toward its goal, developing a team that capitalizes on the unique contributions of team members in a way that complements the individual differences of team members, and managing the many challenges to team effectiveness that arise from both outside and inside of the team.

7

Training Staff: *The Critical Skill for Strategic Managers*

Because of its scientific roots and the pace of change in its technical disciplines, the health care industry has long recognized the importance of training and development. In health care, development is traditionally confined to narrowly circumscribed technical skills such as nursing, anesthesiology, or administration. It is also typically a process mediated by the individual employee, with minimal input from the manager, whose only function is to ensure that the cost of development does not exceed established allotments for an individual cost center.

Organizations with solid records of excellence and innovation, as well as those that have engineered "miraculous" turnarounds in health care and many other industries, however, have adopted a view of training and development that represents a paradigm shift for many managers: an organizational performance system. In this system, employee performance is not simply a function of adequate training and appropriate motivation. It is a function of training, education, job experiences, feedback systems, environmental design, and many other variables.

In this performance system, the manager is a manager not of people but of performance results. The role of the manager in this system is to plan and manage the growth of her staff in such a way that they are not only ready to perform their immediate job tasks but also are constantly preparing for new responsibilities and career moves within the organization. Although this is an exciting and dynamic system for anyone to be a part of, it can be understandably frightening for the manager. Greatly expanded managerial accountability for things that in the past have been the jobs of the training department or management development presents many challenges for managers. For those who accept these challenges, however, this responsibility is accompanied with great rewards. Among them are increased competence, productivity, and job satisfaction among staff and greater recognition and personal job satisfaction for the manager. This chapter will present a rationale for aggressively managing employee development as a competitive weapon. It will focus on the manager's planning function in training and in more broadly focused employee development. Practical strategies within an overall management approach are presented. I will discuss briefly several modalities for providing training, but this will not be my focus for two reasons: (1) Most communities have instructional systems design experts who can advise the manager about delivery strategies and (2) available technologies are growing more numerous every month. The emergence of cost-effective videodisc, hypertext, hypermedia, and many other exciting technologies make the choice of a delivery medium one best managed on a case-by-case basis. Chapter Eight will address tools for expanding our definition of performance improvement to address ways other than training for the manager to enhance individual employee and overall department performance.

Training and development, referred to politely as continuing professional development, is an expensive proposition for the health care provider. Although many providers in the past have supported employee development, the continuation of this support is threatened by pressure on managers to invest their capital in those areas providing substantial returns to the organization's performance. This pressure is often cited by managers and administrators as a reason for reducing the investment made in training and development.

Yet it is precisely because of this pressure to provide performance returns that competitive leaders invest heavily in the development of their employees. Fred Smith, the CEO of Federal Express, has called training "far and away the most important — and best — investment" Federal Express makes. He also puts his money where his mouth is. In 1987–1988, the company spent over $20 million developing a modern training system. Federal Express is currently one of the most successful companies in any industry in the nation. This did not happen with management making heavy investments in needless overhead. Smith, and management leaders like him, expect and get a return on their investment in training and development. Smith went on to explain that the total annual return on his $20 million investment is expected to be in the neighborhood of $120 million. How can such returns be possible, and how can managers achieve them?

To realize the performance returns of training and development, training must be aggressively directed by line managers, rather than allowed to languish through benign neglect or delegation to employees and an "Office of Continuing Education." Delegation of training will result in training that meets only the needs and interests of the employee, not the organization. If one wants to meet the needs of *only* the employee, other strategies, among them a vacation, are effective. Training is not, I repeat, *not* an employee benefit. It is a job requirement.

To ensure that the requirement for training is met, successful organizations hold line managers accountable for its delivery and subsequent job application. Arthur Andersen & Co., one of the largest consulting firms in the world, requires that its managers deliver all training. There are several truths about training and development that must be kept in mind by managers at all levels of the organization.

- Training and development is an investment in an organization's competitive position.
- Performance expectations to be achieved from employee development must be clearly stated and quantitatively measured.

- Employees and managers must be held accountable for performance in training and development, as in all other areas of job performance.
- Managers must know how to supervise training and development.

The Six Faces of Training

To manage employee training and development, health care managers must understand the total scope of that training. Effective training and development address six performance needs in a balanced manner. These six performance areas reflect both the needs of the employee and those of the manager's organization in three distinct areas of skill. The six areas are shown in Figure 7.1.

Planning must be done to develop employee skills for two very different sets of performance needs, as indicated by the left side of the matrix in Figure 7.1. The first of these are the needs of the organization. An example of these needs might be a need to provide home care services for postsurgical patients. This need has implications for management planning of employee training in technical skill areas, business skill areas, and industry knowledge. The second performance need area is that of the

Figure 7.1. Six Types of Training.

Performance Needs	Technical Skills	Business Skills	Industry Knowledge
Organization	••••	••••	••••
Individual Employee	••••	••••	••••

Note: Dots indicate amount of emphasis in any given area.

individual employee. An example of this might be a nurse who wants to develop skills in neonatal nursing.

To plan for training to meet these performance needs, the manager must consider employee training in three different knowledge areas: technical skills, which are job-specific, business skills, and a conceptual understanding of the health care industry.

Technical skills include the use of an intra-aortic balloon pump (including associated physiology and pathology) for nurses and planning implications of the Health Care Finance Administration regulation changes for the CEO and director of marketing.

Business skills include behavioral skills of management as well as analytical skills, such as financial management. These skills are almost nonexistent at the level of supervisor and department manager in many provider organizations. This is due largely to the professional roots of managers and promotion without preparation by health care organizations.

Industry knowledge is the awareness of and ability to monitor and evaluate development of trends in the health care system. These trends are in service delivery systems (HMOs), medical science, and regulation and management of the industry. This knowledge is critical to effective planning and job performance at all levels of the organization. Industry knowledge must be systematically developed in every organizational level, from the board to nonexempt personnel.

Continuing professional development in health care often (though not always) focuses on issues of technical importance to a specific group of specialists. Such an exclusive focus neglects five other performance areas and creates a matrix like the one in Figure 7.2.

Tens of thousands of dollars may be spent on training and professional development in an organization, yet its performance needs remain largely unmet, as do the business skills and industry knowledge development needs of the individual employee. This matrix is a generalization. The exact portrait of training will vary from person to person and department to department, but the weighted trend in development will be the

Figure 7.2 Traditional Training Emphasis in Health Care.

Performance Needs	Technical Skills	Business Skills	Industry Knowledge
Organization	•		
Employee	• • • •		•

same. The first goal of managing development in staff is to achieve a balance in the training provided so that the investment made in training meets organizational and individual performance needs in all three areas.

How does a manager solve this problem? The soundest approach first considers the performance goals of the organization and the department and uses these as a foundation to identify training priorities. Following this general approach, the manager will build a model that ensures an acceptable return on the training and development dollar. This model requires an analysis of department performance needs, assessment of group and individual competencies among staff, and, finally, one-on-one planning with staff members to build an individual development plan matching a person's needs and career interests with the department's priorities. Figure 7.3 shows this relationship between organizational performance and effective training. This approach, which moves from the general importance of organizational goals to specific planning priorities for staff development, requires four steps.

1. Review the strategic plan priorities for the entire organization to determine overall performance priorities. Concentrate on determining the implications of the plan for the departments for which training is to be managed. Consider how it will affect the services offered and its implications for technical, business, and industry knowledge requirements for staff. Often,

Figure 7.3. Organizational Goals as Foundation for Training.

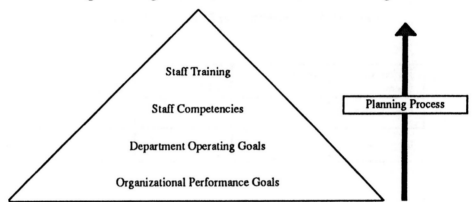

the strategic plan's priorities and operational implications of those priorities can be determined quickly through meetings with administrative officers and the manager's immediate superior.

2. Develop a specific set of leadership issues for the department from the strategic direction of the organization and department. These issues should be developed in conjunction with staff supervisors, using group process techniques to develop a consensus.

3. Develop a profile for department staff in each of the three areas of performance. To do this, the manager must first determine the competencies the staff need to have to achieve the objectives of the operating plan. A sample competency profile is included in the resources section at the back of the book as Resource A: Competency Areas for Health Care Managers. Because this competency listing is for managers, the technical skills listed are actually business skills. The competency profile itself will then be evaluated by supervisors who will assess overall department performance in each competency area. A three-point weighting system is convenient:

- Needs improvement: 1 point
- Adequate: 2 points
- Outstanding (masters): 3 points

Finally, managers will weight each competency in terms of its importance for achievement of department goals. This scale will award points as follows: Critical competencies or those that are new to the staff (for example, marketing or customer service skills) receive 1 point, important competencies receive 2 points, and helpful competencies receive 3 points. By multiplying the weight and performance scores, the manager can focus development planning on those areas of the department performance receiving the lowest total scores. A sample worksheet for determining the hierarchy of competencies to be developed is provided in Resource B at the back of the book.

4. Establish individual development plans for each staff member. This is a process that flows naturally from and into the performance appraisal function. Using as its core the competencies developed earlier, the development plan serves as both a performance management tool and a record of employee strengths and weaknesses to be improved.

Using a top-down approach that systematically assesses both individual development needs and the performance needs of the organization will help ensure that the manager's training dollars are well spent on strategic performance needs. This model is shown in Figure 7.4. Resource D at the back of the book provides an example of this process at work, along with specific steps followed by a manager in a hospital.

The Individual Development Plan

According to the sample development plan in Resource C at the back of the book, there are five critical components to any effective plan:

- Descriptive information about the employee
- A joint employee/supervisory assessment of the employee's performance in department competencies
- An analysis of unique employee assets that can be tapped to the benefit of the department and the staff member

Step

1. Define strategic priorities.
- For organization.
- Implications for department.
- For department operation.

2. Determine impact of performance plans on competencies needed in staff.

3. Evaluate actual versus required level and type of staff competencies.

4. Develop, implement and monitor individual development contracts with staff.

Information Sources

- CEO/COO/administrative officer for department
- Strategic plan for department or division

- Department operating plan
- Department managers, supervisors, and staff

- Supervisory assessment
- Analysis of department performance appraisals

- Individual staff members
- Supervisors
- Performance appraisals
- Operational and management information indicators

Outputs

- Strategic plan priorities for key performance areas
- Impact of strategic plan upon department

- Key competencies needed in staff
- Ideal competency inventory

- Actual existing competency inventory
- Priorities for competency development

- Operational work plan for staff competency development with:
  - Specific development experiences
  - Timetable for implementation
  - Staff accountability for job use of competencies

- A specific development work plan for the employee that focuses on unique strengths and competency needs of the individual
- An assessment of personal ambitions of the employee and how management can support those ambitions

The first of these components is general descriptive information about an employee. This information should include at least the formal education or professional preparation, the length of employment with the health care provider, various positions held with the provider, and a record of all training taken while at the organization. This record should note both external training, such as professional conventions and seminars, and interorganizational training, such as teleconferences, in-service education, and technical training provided by medical products companies on site. All records of training completed should include a statement that summarizes what the employee can do as a result of the training. I recommend this as a minimal level of documentation because more reliable evaluations are often unavailable. Many training programs *claim* to be criterion referenced and competency based but lack the rigorous design necessary to test these claims. With this narrative in a training record, the manager has at least a general understanding of the talent an employee has gained, if not empirical proof of that talent.

This descriptive information about the employee also contains a section to document any significant and potentially important skills that are unique to the staff member. These skills, which might include talents as varied as fund raising and computer programming, can prove valuable to the department and to the growth of the employee. Consider, for example, a hospital's electrical maintenance supervisor who had a background in computer programming in an earlier career in the military. This supervisor was able to provide design and programming support for several projects developing automated management tracking and planning tools for departments in the hospital, saving the cost of hiring external personnel and, in several cases, improving the overall output of department managers. The supervisor was able to apply his unique skills among the hospital staff and gain visibility and recognition from administrators.

This descriptive record is important to the development plan because it tells a manager the investment already made in the employee by the organization and the likelihood of the manager seeing a return of improved performance with any future investment. Employees who are with any single department for only a short time before they transfer to other areas are not strong candidates for specialized training and development at the expense of a department's budget.

The second element in a strong development plan is the employee's analysis of which of the departmental competencies are most important for successful performance and his evaluation of how well he performs at all department competencies. This section also contains the employee's supervisor's opinions regarding the same factors. The supervisor's analysis has been formed over time, through observation of the employee and through performance coaching and appraisal. Indeed, performance appraisals are valuable information sources for supervisors in this phase of development planning.

This joint analysis of competencies forces the supervisor and staff to discuss performance priorities and the causes of any discrepancies in the analysis of an employee's performance. Such discussion is in itself a useful development experience for both parties. Staff members and supervisors often have differing perceptions about the cause of any performance issue. The competency inventory also serves as a foundation for prioritizing development efforts for the employee. High-priority, low-performance competency areas clearly come before growth experiences in employee development.

Another important component of the development plan is a narrative summary by the employee's manager or supervisor of the personal, technical, and managerial assets that the employee brings to her position. This narrative becomes a useful focus for building job experiences within the employee's current position that allow her to capitalize upon those strengths. Clearly this is an important avenue for increasing the value of an employee to a department and rewarding an employee when promotion or financial avenues are not feasible. This can mean either expanding or delimiting the focus of the employee's position to the benefit of both the department and the individual. One example of this was a respiratory therapist who was noted by her supervisor as having very solid coaching and training skills in preoperative education classes for open-heart surgery patients. Through discussion of development planning for the therapist, the supervisor elected to expand the therapist's role to include responsibility for coaching and evaluating all students who rotated through the hospital for clinical training. Another example was the selection of a nurse who had experience as a MASH officer in Vietnam to manage the nursing support for a helicopter medical transport team for a regional trauma center.

Mapping a specific work plan for employee development is the fourth component of a solid development plan. An effective development work plan must specify four critical factors to clarify expectations for employee training and to ensure accountability for performance:

1. Development needs to be addressed by the employee: To be most useful, these needs should be expressed as the specific competencies for department success that the employee will strengthen with the support of her managers.
2. Specific development activities planned for the employee to build each cited competency: Some development needs may require a single experience, while more complex competencies may require several different types of experiences to raise performance to needed levels. A brief treatment of traditional and more innovative options for this development follows this section.
3. Planned job application of developed competencies: Specific contracts for job application increase the likelihood that employees will actually transfer new skills to their daily work routine, and they provide a motivation for the employee to complete planned development activities.
4. A timetable for completion of each development plan component: The timetable will help the manager plan develop-

ment expenses for budgeting department expenses, and it will also serve as a benchmark to track progress for the employee and his supervisor.

An assessment of employee development accomplishments to date will help track ongoing progress and provide an opportunity for the manager to gather useful feedback from the staff regarding the effectiveness of both internal and external training investments. Next, the development plan must consider the longer-range issues of career positioning and responsibility of importance to the individual staff member. To be considered in this phase of development planning are the employee's ambitions and his supervisor's recommendations regarding feasible alternatives to accomplish those ambitions.

If there is any reasonable way for department management to support the long-term development of the employee by providing skills or experience that will prepare the employee for career positioning, it should be planned and recorded in the development plan. Frequently effective options for this are special assignments outside the department or responsibility for a project that is important to the department and provides an opportunity for an employee's talent to be recognized by a broader community in the organization. In departments where such opportunities are not available, managers may elect to systematically cross-train high-potential staff in multiple areas of expertise. This is not only intelligent staff development but also very helpful to managers when staffing shortages threaten department effectiveness.

Practical Strategies for Staff Development

This section describes several of the many strategies available to the health care manager to deliver training and development to staff. This list is far from exhaustive, but it does cover several representative strategies and criteria for effectively using them.

Traditional In-Service Education

Traditionally structured in-service education can be very effective for developing technical knowledge. It generally should not be used to develop behavioral skills because the classroom or laboratory structure and typically short duration of in-service education do not allow the practice and feedback necessary for effective development of these skills.

To be successful, in-service education should focus on those topics that are recent developments in a specific technical area, reviews of currently known but seldom used information (for example, the diagnosis and treatment protocol for Reye's Syndrome), or new to the staff but which naturally build on its technical foundation (for example, the pharmacology of a newly introduced cardioactive drug to critical care nurses). In-service education must occur at regular intervals, no less frequently than monthly. Participation should be mandatory for all staff members. This creates minor logistical problems in departments that are staffed twenty-four hours a day. These problems are best resolved by conducting the in-service education on each shift or using a videocassette recorder and camera.

Department staff should be responsible for planning each in-service event. Faculty can be identified by staff and management and recruited from medical or administrative staff and schools with which the hospital has affiliations. In general, the department manager should select in-service faculty. One effective option for staff development is to regularly use staff members to research and deliver in-service training to peers.

Internal Management Skill Development

Internal development of management skills can be effective in preparing select staff members for roles as supervisors and managers. The components of a program of internal development of management skills include a desire on the part of the manager and staff member to move the staff member away from technical responsibilities and into a supervisory role over a period of time. This might seem to be silly, but to many allied health professionals, the idea of replacing the practice of their medical support skills with "administrivia" is not a pleasant one, even if a pay raise is attached. Also needed is a development plan that specifies classroom development of management skills in analytical functions (for example, budgeting and determining staffing patterns) and behavioral skills (conflict resolution, negotiation, and coaching, for example). Finally, on-the-job preparation is essential, including assignment to a supervisor/manager for observation and then actual rotation through each of the supervisory jobs; during these rotations an incumbent supervisor gives performance feedback to the trainee.

External Seminars

External seminars are those provided to staff personnel by organizations or consultants from outside the health care organization. Seminars are different from in-service education in that they are longer (generally at least half a day) and focus upon developing a broader knowledge base about a single performance issue.

External seminars have several advantages for the manager and participating staff. They have the potential to present often unexpected and beneficial exchanges of ideas through in-class discussion with participants from other hospitals and other areas of the country. Many staff members see them as an opportunity to "get away" from the routine of work and to grow professionally. Employees often take a certain pride in the knowledge that management values them because it is willing to spend the money to send them to an off-site seminar.

The greatest problem for the manager using the external seminar for staff development is quality assurance. The real training value of many continuing education seminars, particularly those in the behavioral skills areas, is questionable. This is because seminar leaders focus upon entertaining rather than educating participants. This does not mean that seminars must be boring. Quite the contrary—they should be engaging to the learner without being distracting. However, this distinction is lost on some seminar faculty. The manager's recourse in quality assurance is to use available information to evaluate each seminar before writing the tuition and hotel checks for the staff. This can be done by reading promotional material for the program, requesting a review of participant manuals for the program, and asking the opinion of prior participants in the seminar. Here are a few things to look for as quality indicators. Besides checking the credentials of the faculty or sponsoring organization, ask two questions:

1. Are there specific objectives that the learner will accomplish as a result of the seminar? These should clearly tell the manager precisely what her staff person will be able to do on the job after the seminar that is different from what he can presently do at work. The manager can then determine whether this change is appropriate and important enough to the department to warrant payment. If there are no objectives for a specific seminar and none can be divined after contacting faculty, then the quality of the program is suspect.

2. Are the teaching methods used in the seminar really going to develop the skills in staff members that are stated in the objectives? If not, then the staff member may learn a lot about a topic, but his performance may not change noticeably. There are well-established and generally accepted guidelines for how to build different types of skills in adults. Failure to follow these guidelines because of time constraints is the most common reason for the failure of behavioral skill development. It is impossible to have any significant effect on a person's ability to resolve conflict, negotiate, coach, or speak effectively in public through lecture-intensive seminars with little or no practice.

Professional Symposia/Conferences

Professional symposia and association conferences have several benefits for both the staff member and the department that are very different from those offered by a seminar. These benefits include providing a condensed survey of recent developments and industry issues as they affect the department's profession. Conferences allow a person to quickly learn about developments in many areas of the nation and many specialties of a given discipline. From this survey, the staff member may find useful ideas for the performance of the department. These ideas are different from and complementary to the development of specific skills developed in more thorough treatments of any issue or skill area. Additionally, association conferences often contain working sessions at which a staff member will have an opportunity to participate and influence the future direction of the professional association. In this way, the development needs of the staff constituency are represented to the association and considered in the planning of future credentialing, development, and lobbying functions of the professional association.

Computer-Supported Training

Personal computers (PCs) can effectively deliver both information and technical skill training in a variety of formats. In recent years, PC-based training for allied health and business skill development has exploded in content and variety of media available.

There are many sources for information about available training in computer-based formats. Among the best are specific professional societies for the various professions, the American Health Association and its affiliate organizations, and client education support from computer manufacturers. The latter group can generally provide a manager with a listing of many vendors and developers of computer-based training (CBT) and development specifically related to a particular subject.

With the tremendous expansion in available CBT programs also comes a tremendous expansion in poor-quality CBT. The manager who would evaluate CBT must ask the following questions:

- Is the intended target audience for the program the same as your staff?
- Are there specific performance objectives that a user should be able to accomplish after the training?
- Does the program make effective use of graphics, questioning, testing, and other strategies to engage the user in a meaningful way?
- Can the user review material in the program on demand?

Management Development Internships

The continued development of a high-potential staff supervisor frequently is best served by temporarily removing that person from the mainstream of department activities. A management development internship involves rotating a supervisor through diverse operating areas as an assistant to their managers for project assignments. The internship is useful for developing a broader perspective of the scope and business of health care in the staff person. A richer understanding of the contributions made by other departments in the hospital is generally the outcome of such a rotation.

This enrichment in turn enriches the department in that the supervisor will learn how other departments are managed and bring that knowledge back to the department after the rotation. A solid understanding of the diverse functions of a health care provider will change the supervisor by breaking the bonds of professional parochialism (the "us versus them" mindset), which is frequently evident in professional departments of a hospital.

Solo Project Management Responsibility

Solo project management provides an opportunity for the manager to leverage research and development and to delegate administrative projects effectively. Staff members assigned project management responsibility can develop project management skills, use personal strengths and talents, and in many cases achieve more prominent organizational visibility. There is another benefit of this for both the staff member and management.

One of the greatest threats to staffing levels among allied health professionals is burnout created by a high-stress environ-ment, routine protocol for managing human crises, and a lack of professional autonomy. (See Chapter Six.) In the hospital, while most allied health professionals can have input into patient care on treatment decisions, only physical therapists and a handful of others have the autonomy to make independent decisions about optimum patient care protocol.

Often assigning a staff member to manage a significant project for the department can address these performance needs as well as those of the department. Staff members should not, however, be selected for special project work based upon proximity to impending burnout. Selection should be based on the individual talents of the staff member, unique personal attributes, and their interest in the project. Candidates for spe-cial projects can be screened by reviewing individual develop-ment plans for staff personnel.

These are only some of the avenues open to the effective health care manager in developing her staff. They vary in cost and cover a wide variety of different development needs. Others that have been effectively used in health care organizations include cross-training staff in a progressively broader scope of job functions, research and development of service lines offered by the department, assignment to adjunct faculty responsibili-ties, and mentorship.

Management Skill Development in Health Care

The development of management competencies is a spe-cial challenge for the management leader in health care. The managerial leader must ensure that the highly individualized management skill development needs of all supervisors and managers who report to her are met. In addition, the manager must also actively assess and plan the development of her own skills.

The health care manager who has a professional background in one of the many technical disciplines of health care has a special need for management skill development. The professional preparation of this manager has likely emphasized one or more of the pure sciences and extensive medical application of those sciences. Rarely does this manager come into his position with any solid development of management skills. The manager has probably had some exposure to the general management process or to management issues as they affect health care delivery. And many managers have had several courses surveying management functions. But true skill development is rarely achieved without detailed study of specific competencies and extensive practice with expert feedback at the application of those skills.

The management skills important to health care managers are the same as those important to other industries. These skills fall into three broad areas:

- Analytical and financial skills
- Behavioral skills for effective management of people
- Decision-making and risk-taking skills

For the health care manager these are the technical skills to which I referred in the treatment of the six faces of management. The health care manager is a management specialist first and a technical expert second.

Many tools are available to the health care manager to help him determine the talents and development needs in both his staff and himself. But before using these tools, the manager should know what general areas of management skill are going to be most important for any given managerial role. The success of the frontline supervisor is critically dependent upon mastery of the "soft skills" of people management. These include coaching, identifying performance problems, counseling, resolving conflicts, and negotiating. Analytical skills and related problem solving are crucial for the midlevel manager responsible for one or more departments. At the level of senior executive, skills at people management and analytical management techniques should already be in place. The challenge for these managers is

Figure 7.5. Relative Need for Different Management Skills.

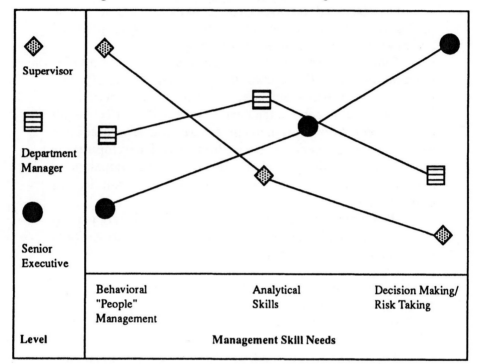

to develop the problem-solving and risk-taking skills needed to position an entire organization to have a vision for quality health care and competitive advantage at the same time.

Figure 7.5 demonstrates the extent to which managers at different levels in an organization rely on different types of management skills. As the figure shows, the success of a senior executive relies less on supervisory skills inherent to behavioral management and more on the judgment required for making effective organizational decisions and taking appropriate business risks.

Each person brings to management a unique set of talents and development needs. Many supervisors will have as a priority the development of management behavioral skills, but there may well be many who have mastered many of these skills and would be better served by strengthening their analytical skills of service planning and financial management. This raises the first major issue of management skill development for self and staff. How do you objectively determine what needs to be developed in whom?

Assessing Management Development Needs

There are many approaches to assessing management talent. One approach assesses a manager with feedback from the staff regarding their observations of management skill. Many of the assessment tools using this approach often include two components: a written survey designed to gather information about performance in key areas and a critical incident reporting tool to cite empirical evidence of a specific level of skill.

One useful method of gathering information about the behavioral management skills that need to be developed in a department is to ask managers and the people who report to them to independently complete the same questionnaire about the manager's strengths and development needs. Aside from the manager, these questionnaires should remain anonymous and be returned to the manager's immediate superior or training planner. Determine the average and range of scores for the manager's performance as reported by staff and compare them with the manager's self-report. Areas with a high level of consistency between the manager's self-report and the aggregate of his direct reports indicate clear development needs. Areas in which the manager's report indicates a solid skill level, yet which are inconsistent with the staff's report, will require comparison with the assessment by the manager's immediate superior or development counseling with the manager to determine likely causes for the discrepancy and discussion of the possibility of training.

I am only recommending the use of staff evaluation of managerial strengths to assess training needs. I do *not* support the concept of employee evaluations of their manager for purposes of managerial performance appraisal. That is the responsibility of the manager's immediate superior.

Staff evaluation of managers has been attempted in health care in recent years, in part as an attempt to develop in all employees an appreciation for "customer orientation." Although this is conceptually appealing, in practice it has proven terribly unreliable and in some cases destructive. In one large Midwestern hospital, this practice was instituted at the same time that management was reviewing the performance of all employees in preparation for restructuring and reducing staff. The staffs of several very effective and supportive managers evaluated their managers very poorly, due in large part to the managers' attempts to encourage higher levels of productivity and work quality from their staffs (potentially to save their jobs). Because managerial performance appraisals had been redesigned to heavily weight the input of these disgruntled employees, these managers' ratings suffered. As a result, the hospital lost two of these managers and kept in their employ staff who resisted much needed and reasonable improvements to work quality.

This is not meant as a condemnation of the practice of subordinate input into managerial evaluations. Rather, it is a caution to monitor the implementation of such practices carefully. In any assessment, but particularly when structured to include input from subordinates, the evaluative process must consider the entire scope of managerial responsibility, including those that are invisible to staff and therefore beyond the realm of their meaningful critique.

Assessing managers' needs for analytical skill development is most easily accomplished by determining the prior training of a manager in quantitative management areas and the present and short-term future needs for these skills in the manager's position. In many cases, supervisors and managers in health care have had little training in developing or interpreting the operational importance of a budget or in determining the financial feasibility of service development, much less any of the more complex skills of financial management. What typically happens in health care at this level of management is quick on-the-job training from people who themselves may have shaky skills. This is not enough to succeed in health care management in the twenty-first century.

An effective alternative to this, albeit somewhat more intimidating for the manager, is to take one of many criterion-referenced tests of management skills in the quantitative competencies. An advantage to testing is precision in determining the manager's strengths and weaknesses in the areas of quantitative competence. A disadvantage of testing is cost, which can range from $70 to $350 per manager/supervisor assessed. It may be wiser to rely upon a review of prior training and the manager's self-assessment of skill in the area. A review of the American College of Healthcare Executives Membership Examination for the years 1985–1987 showed that the average score of all candidates for membership status in this prestigious organization was under 67 percent (Stevens, 1987b). Given this, it is a safe training and development bet to assume that any given manager without at least a bachelor's degree in business or ten years of job experience would benefit from financial skills training.

What Is Good Management Skill Training?

The quality of management skill training is determined largely by how it is delivered to the managers. By this I do not mean the name recognition factor or the entertainment skills of the faculty. There are several critical attributes of effective management skill training, which are particular to the skills for handling people, finances, and decision making.

Effective people management skills must be trained over several days and generally away from the worksite. Such training should emphasize practice and hands-on experimentation for the audience. This practice must be augmented by feedback from a competent trainer. One frequent mistake in the design of training of this type for managers is that it focuses on making the theoretical aspects of behavioral science understandable in layperson's terms. This is typically done with entertaining anecdotes and clever mnemonics. In reality, managers and supervisors need little of the theory of behavioral science. What they do need is practice and practice and more practice at applying concrete skills. Only through this practice in simulated job situations will people skills ever be engrained in the daily routine of staff management. This training should have a component that the manager and his staff or direct superior can use to help the manager transfer the skills by applying them at work. Interpersonal skills are impossible to develop adequately in a single program or even curriculum. These skills must be developed, reviewed, and practiced always.

Effective training for financial and quantitative skills must present reasons or principles, as well as technical aspects, so the manager can use the skills in a variety of situations back at work. The training should focus on applying the principles and skills in case studies and simulations that begin with routine job situations, but quickly move beyond this to new applications within the confines of business management. This will help the manager to see the universal applicability of the quantitative principles and encourage their application in a wide variety of work contexts. Also helpful are tools such as computer diskettes, decision-making guides, flow charts, references, and other job aids that the manager can use to apply the skills back in the hospital.

Finally, effective training for decision making and risk taking must provide opportunities for managers to apply existing skills in new situations, where there is no one right answer. Such training should allow managers to compare the effectiveness of their decision making to that of peers from other departments or hospitals. It should also allow managers the freedom to make mistakes and successful decisions without fear of retribution, ridicule, or discipline. The manager must be able to witness the effect of her decisions and to explore the dynamics between the case problems at hand and the decisions she made.

How Big an Investment?

There is no one right answer to the question of how much a manager should budget for training and development of staff. The size of the investment must be determined individually, after consideration of the ambition of organizational strategy, existing competence of the department, time frames for achieving performance goals, and the cost/benefit of using technologically advanced alternatives to traditional training.

There are, however, a few basic rules of thumb:

- The average successful American company invests 1.2 percent of its total employee payroll costs (including an average of 26 percent of base costs for employee benefits) in training and development. The range is from .2 percent to 3.6 percent.
- In general, it is less expensive to buy prepackaged training from vendors than to create it through custom development. There is, however, a trade-off in such savings. Very few "canned" vendor training programs are as effective in creating the performance improvement accomplished with training custom designed by specialists.
- In general, training technical skills is easier and quicker than training the behavioral skills of management. Behavioral skills are generally more complex and require much greater effort by the manager to force practice and on-the-job application of behavioral skills.

Summary

The department manager must manage the training and development of staff as aggressively as operational and financial determinants of department success. When properly managed, training of staff is an investment in the organization's competitive position. Training and development also increase the value of the individual employee to the organization and improve morale and job satisfaction among staff.

Effective management of staff training requires a planning process that begins with an examination of the strategic direction of the health care organization and the implications of that direction for department performance needs. From this general starting point, the manager must define the competencies needed in department staff to meet performance

challenges, evaluate existing performance levels in these competency areas, and develop a focus for staff training and development. Finally, the manager and supervisors of the department
must work with each staff member to develop, implement, and
monitor the progress of individual development plans.

These development plans serve as a central intelligence
file of sorts, detailing the training and talents of the employee
and providing a work plan for continued development. The
development plan serves to ensure accountability of the individual employee for completing and applying on the job any
training that a manager's budget supports.

8

Managing Staff Performance:
Monitoring, Feedback, and Reinforcement

Among the greatest challenges that health care managers face are continual staff turnover, burnout, and limited resources and the fluctuations in performance quality that they create. There is much advice available to managers in factories and other production-oriented businesses about ways to manage these issues. When health care managers attempt to follow this advice, they find that they face situations unique to the provider organization. Many approaches to performance improvement that are effective in a widget factory simply do not work in a health care environment. This is unfortunate because nowhere in American industry is performance more important, and nowhere in industry is the need to "do more with less" a greater imperative.

Traditional approaches to performance improvement do not translate to health care primarily because of the autonomous nature of the work and the highly professional environment of the provider. The very act of monitoring work performance creates special difficulties for the health care manager. How does one accurately assess and improve the performance of staff that are spread out over a ward, a floor, or an entire institution? This chapter will present principles and tools for effective performance improvement in health care provider organizations.

The Components of Performance

What distinguishes a high-performing department, staff, or manager from one that is mediocre or poor? It is the ability to not only meet but also exceed basic performance expectations on a consistent basis. For the high performer, status quo is not good enough. Anyone who has worked in health care delivery has seen individual staff members who are highly motivated and seem always to give 110 percent. They have also seen staff members who arrive five minutes before a shift is to begin and leave precisely at the end of that shift. If a patient report is needed, these people will dash off a brief written summary and leave it for the incoming shift, rather than spend the time needed to provide detailed oral reports on patients' conditions. The trick for the health care manager is to systematically build an entire staff that gives 110 percent, 100 percent of the time.

Effective performance management has been proven to increase the quantity and quality of department and company output by as much as 500 percent (Daniels and Rosen, 1984). Beyond this, performance management has been shown to produce many spin-off benefits of special interest to health care managers. Among these are reductions in employee turnover and greatly improved staff morale. To realize this improvement in performance, a manager must build two elements into the management structure of a department. The first of these is a performance improvement infrastructure. A prerequisite to managing performance improvement, this infrastructure consists of clearly defined expectations for all job functions and effective performance goals. The second element is the management process needed to achieve and maintain superior achievement. Altogether, the manager must build a system of six components:

- *Comprehensive performance expectations for all job components.* This, in the minds of many managers, is why department policy and procedure manuals exist. To be effective as a management tool, however, the procedure manual must state expectations in terms of specific behaviors and be in daily use by managers and staff alike and not archived in the department head's office in a locked cabinet.

- *Relevant, measurably stated performance goals for individuals, shifts, and an entire department.* These goals are different from the performance expectations in procedure manuals. Performance goals are broader in scope and deal with issues of customer service.

- *Quantifiable measures* of baseline or current performance levels relative to those indicated in performance goals.

- *Regular and frequent feedback* from managers to staff. This feedback must be reinforcing rather than punishing. It must be designed to make staff *want* to improve performance and tell them *how* to improve performance.

- *Positive reinforcement* administered at times that will best sustain any improvements in performance.

- *A data-based system for monitoring* detailed and ongoing performance empirically.

Performance Infrastructure

Performance Expectations

In most provider organizations, the Joint Committee for Accreditation of Healthcare Organizations mandates require a complete listing of all procedures that staff job functions encompass. This requirement ensures that the department has clearly stated performance expectations—or does it? To perform effectively on the job, most clinicians must be skilled in three areas: (1) A thorough knowledge of the scientific or theoretical base for their work, (2) application of that knowledge consistent with the procedural documentation of a department, and (3) communication with and support of clients (usually patients and their families). It would not do at all for a nurse to understand the collected works of Kübler-Ross and yet be unable to communicate with and support a terminally ill patient. Similarly, a therapist who knows how to assemble equipment and administer treatment would be dangerous if she were unable to determine the cause of an adverse reaction to treatment because she was a little shaky on her pharmacology. Because of these additional dimensions of performance, existing procedure manuals probably are insufficient to use as a tool for performance improvement.

How then, can a manager develop performance expectations that address the theory and communication dimensions of performance as well as the practice/procedure dimension? Criterion-referenced performance standards that address all components of performance are effective for this need. To develop these standards, expand upon (or if need be, develop) comprehensive procedural statements like those in a procedure manual. This expansion must build into existing procedures the span of knowledge and communication skills needed for accurate performance of each job task or procedure. In developing these standards, establish observable indicators of the use of communicative and knowledge skills.

For example, a performance standard for providing care to a patient would certainly expect that the care giver would communicate with the patient to minimize the patient's anxiety and elicit his or her cooperation with any procedure. As stated, however, that performance expectation is nebulous and subject to interpretation in a number of ways.

If, however, the performance expectation is referenced to commonly accepted performance criteria, it becomes much easier to measure. These criteria are observable indicators of that communication. For example, observable criteria for effective communication might include: "The care giver will identify himself or herself to the patient by name and department" and "The care giver will explain the therapy procedure, rationale, and effect upon the patient, verifying the patient's understanding with questions." In most provider institutions, it is commonly accepted that this communication will put a patient at ease and foster cooperation. When there are obvious reasons for a criterion to be waived it can be relaxed. For example, when caring for an unconscious patient, it is impossible to verify the patient's understanding but not impossible to identify oneself to the patient.

The power of specific criteria for performance expecta-

Exhibit 8.1. Criterion Checklist for Performance Feedback.

Performance Requirements: Physical Therapy

Criterion	Yes	No	Comment
1. Dons protective surgical gloves before entering patient room.			
2. Identifies patient by ID bracelet.			
3. Introduces self to patient.			
4. Explains purpose of visit.			
5. Explains benefits of procedure to be administered.			

tions lies in the ability of a manager to pinpoint desired behavior and provide precise feedback about staff performance. One practical method for employing performance criteria is to include them in an observation checklist that includes each criterion for a procedure, a check-box that any observer can use to indicate successful performance of a criterion, and room for documenting qualitative notes for feedback to a staff member (see Exhibit 8.1).

Performance Goals

When performance goals are properly developed and communicated, they provide a relevant target for the staff. In addition, properly constructed goals provide increased opportunity for managers to provide feedback and positive reinforcement for staff members' performance growth. The importance of this opportunity cannot be overstated. To improve staff performance for prolonged periods, a manager must provide supportive feedback about performance and reinforce staff for any improvements in performance. This has been repeatedly demonstrated in research studies around the nation. The most commonly used management tools, money and criticism, are ineffective at improving performance. They create only short-term improvements in performance or help extinguish undesirable (and sometimes desirable) behaviors.

An effective performance goal focuses upon customer service and departmental performance issues, as opposed to procedural performance. For example, procedural specification, taken from the procedure manual of a Dietary and Food Services department, might provide detailed performance expectations for what must be done to properly deliver a patient's meal after preparation. A performance goal for the same department might set as a target "delivering all meals to the entire patient population in an average of fifteen minutes from the time they are prepared." The difference between the goal and the procedure is one of customer satisfaction and departmental performance. The performance goal also should include a quantifiable measure of desired performance and any qualifying conditions. This measure should be relevant to overall department performance. The food services goal of fifteen minutes is certainly measurable and relevant to customer satisfaction. Of the customer complaints about institutional food services, lateness and coldness follow poor quality as the most frequent offenses. The goal also includes a qualification—all meals are to be delivered in an average of fifteen minutes—not every single meal. The new wing for geriatric care in this hospital is far from the main kitchen and may require twenty minutes, while most other areas can be served in under fifteen minutes. In addition, a useful performance goal can be divided into component milestones. For example, achieving an average meal delivery of fifteen minutes might not occur in a single week or month, for a variety of reasons. But if past staff performance was thirty-five minutes, and in a week it is down to twenty-five minutes, and a week later, twenty minutes, then significant progress can be observed. There are two reasons for dividing performance goals into component milestones. The first is to allow the manager and staff to monitor actual progress. The second, more important reason is that incremental progress toward a goal

creates opportunity for feedback and reinforcement of performance. This feedback and reinforcement increases the likelihood that effort and performance improvement will continue.
This process is the "magic" of performance management and
often produces performance levels that over time exceed even
an ambitious goal.

Performance Assessment

The final component in building a management infrastructure is the establishment of meaningful measures of
existing levels of staff performance. Baseline performance indicators that are effective provide all staff and managers with a
clear understanding of their overall performance in both quality and quantity of work. Performance measures of this sort are
routine components of many industries and are used to communicate both the challenge of reaching a goal and to demonstrate
relative progress by movement from a baseline toward a goal.
Providers often use the concept of baseline measures in providing care. In rehabilitation, a patient's baseline abilities are assessed prior to starting a therapeutic regimen. Periodically during the treatment regimen, these same values are assessed again,
and improvements are demonstrated to patients. This appraisal
reinforces the patient to make continued effort and continued
improvement.

In the day-to-day world of health care delivery and management, however, the quantity of work performed is generally
viewed as less important than the quality of work performed.
This is especially true at the level of the staff clinical professional
and least consistently observed in administrative and technical
support professions. For example, the number of patients
treated by a physical therapist (on staff) in a given day does not
have the same relevance to him that the number of electrical
installations completed would have for a master electrician. I
differentiate between a staff physical therapist and an independently operating professional for one reason in particular. Staff
professionals who are generally salaried are sheltered from the
need to "generate business" to earn a living. But independently

Table 8.1. Types of Performance Measures for Health Care.

	Technical Quality	Quantity of Work	Customer Satisfaction	Financial Performance
Individual Staff	•	•	•	§
Specialty Teams (Emergency room, for example)	•	•	•	§
Shift	•	•	•	§
Department	•	•	•	•

Key: • Always § If appropriate to work

employed professionals, such as some physical therapists and most physicians, are acutely aware of the fact that more patients translate directly into a larger paycheck. As we move from the infrastructure to the process of performance improvement, I will present techniques a manager may use to help reinforce in staff professionals an understanding and value for monitoring and improving the business and other nonclinical components of care provision. As health professionals come to understand the system of care delivery from a business perspective as well as a scientific and ethical understanding, the differences between staff professionals and independently employed clinicians will be narrowed, but they will nonetheless persist.

What kinds of baseline measures should be developed? This depends entirely upon the department's work and how that department's overall performance is assessed by administrators and clients. In general, performance measures must be developed for the types of performance shown in Table 8.1. In addition to these routine performance indicators, there will frequently develop a need to establish indicators of performance that are unique to the achievement of a particular goal, whether that goal is important to an individual staff member or an entire department.

As mentioned above, the precise type of performance indicator in each of these categories will vary from department to department and perhaps among staff members. It will always be dictated by the nature of the work and performance goals.

A useful starting point for monitoring the technical quality of services provided by staff is to periodically observe performance using criterion-referenced standards to evaluate and provide feedback for performance. A point system can be developed to simplify the process of measuring performance quality.

Quantitative measures of performance present a creative challenge to the health care manager. In the vast majority of provider services, developing a simple widget-counting system for this purpose is inadequate because staff (particularly patient care staff) frequently are given a mix of assignments that vary dramatically in their scope and complexity. After all, performing a portable X ray on a multiple trauma patient in the emergency room is generally much more difficult than performing the same procedure on a person recovering from pneumonia.

This challenge is not insurmountable. The manager must develop a process for reflecting the relationship between service complexity and productivity. For example, in a respiratory care department, a meaningful indicator of the quantity of work might be derived from the total number of treatment procedures performed, multiplied by a complexity factor, to reflect the varying degree of patient support needed. A rehabilitative program for chronic lung disease would likely be more complex in terms of time and patient coaching required than would be monitoring ventilators; a competent therapist could monitor and maintain two or perhaps three mechanical ventilators in the time required to complete one patient visit. A similar structure might apply for assessing baseline nursing staff performance.

Determining baseline customer service and satisfaction measures presupposes a common understanding of who the customers of a department are. This issue is addressed in many marketing texts available and summarized in Chapters Four and Five.

Developing relevant indicators of financial performance may also be a new experience for technically oriented department leaders. This can be done effectively with input from financial officers and administrative superiors. Meeting budget specifications for expenses and income is certainly one indicator, but it is also so global from the perspective of individual staff members as to be meaningless. A key consideration in deciding how and when to use financial indicators of performance is whether the department or staff member has any *direct* impact upon a financial measure of performance. If so, isolate those behaviors that will impact that indicator and express performance goals in terms of that behavior. One simple example of this is the ability of staff members to reduce disposable equipment costs through appropriate use and documentation. A single staff nurse cannot directly tell whether or not she is contributing to cost control for a unit. But she can measure the number of times she accurately charges patient accounts for intravenous setups and fluids. One financial performance indicator that might be established for staff nurses in her unit could focus on that performance, rather than on the dollar value of disposables consumed for the unit.

The Performance Management Process

Thus far we have discussed the importance of managing performance and have identified several components of performance that must be managed. This section presents an overview of the process by which a manager improves performance. This process is a simple one. This can be deceptive, though, because it is as powerful when implemented as it is simple to grasp in concept. The process entails establishing meaningful performance goals for staff and the department, providing feedback on that performance, and reinforcing performance results.

Communicating Performance

All of the defining, monitoring, and analyzing of performance that a manager does will be for nothing unless it serves as a foundation for a continual process of feedback and reinforcement through which improvement can occur. The value of developing quantifiable indicators of goals for performance is that they strengthen the manager's ability to provide feedback on and offer positive reinforcement for staff efforts. The terms *feedback* and *reinforcement* sound like they belong in a behavioral

Figure 8.1. An Overview of Performance Management.

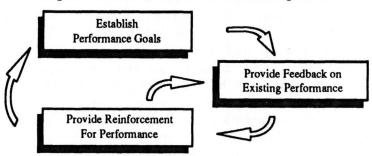

science laboratory rather than a busy workplace. Managers who use these terms often use them interchangeably with the word *communication*. In making this comparison, many would-be performance managers take their first steps on a path to failure.

A manager who is friendly with staff, maintains an open-door policy, or offers frequent "atta-boys" to staff is not necessarily managing performance. And effective feedback is definitely not simple communication. Finally, there is a clear difference between praise and the spectrum of feedback needed to improve performance.

Managing performance seems a straightforward procedure. It is an ongoing cycle of communicating performance goals, providing feedback on current performance levels, and giving positive reinforcement for progress toward goals (see Figure 8.1). The challenge comes in making certain that feedback is effective and reinforcements are meaningful for all staff. If feedback and reinforcement are effective, they encourage improved performance. If they are ineffective, they can actually make staff stop trying to perform. A second challenge for busy managers who would improve total performance is the imperative that this process be repeated again and again until it becomes an automatic response of the manager to daily events.

Having developed important goals for staff performance, the first step in the ongoing journey toward excellence is to clearly communicate those goals to the people who will achieve them. This must be done not just once, but constantly. This repetition is necessary to maintain a continual focus on the importance of those goals in the face of many distractions from issues that arise and compete with focused performance. Among these issues are fluctuating patient care loads, disputes between departments or individuals, and issues unrelated to work that people inevitably bring with them to their jobs. The ability, or lack thereof, to focus on the importance of perfor- mance goals is what distinguishes success from failure in many undertakings beyond the workplace. It is the inability to focus on the importance of physical fitness in the face of exercise pain that sidetracks many a would-be bodybuilder or weight-loss candidate. So too, the ability of the health care manager to focus staff energy on the importance of performance goals is a critical element in obtaining sustained performance growth.

The ways a manager can focus this energy are as varied as the number of health care managers. However, general advice from successful managers of performance includes definition and visualization. First, simplify and summarize goals. It is generally not necessary to deluge a staff with details about how goals have been developed. It is usually adequate to define and communicate the specific goal and its impact upon the patient (or other client), the department, and the staff. Second, commu- nicate visually. Develop and prominently post graphic indica- tors of goal performance and actual current performance (see Figure 8.2). Visual representation of goals is well known to be effective for focusing attention to both the goal and the effort needed to achieve that goal. But if simply making an attractive graph were enough to ensure that communication occurs, the plethora of inspirational posters on department walls and in patient rooms around the nation would be worth their weight in gold. Graphs and other visuals can make a powerful first impres- sion, but that impression can only be maintained through on- going reference to the underlying goal and ensuring that its personal relevance to each staff member is established. A man- ager must incorporate communication of goals with staff mem- bers at every legitimate opportunity: at staff meetings, the change of shifts, in one-on-one meetings and coaching sessions with staff, and at a variety of other times. The way a manager

Figure 8.2. Sample Performance Feedback Graph.

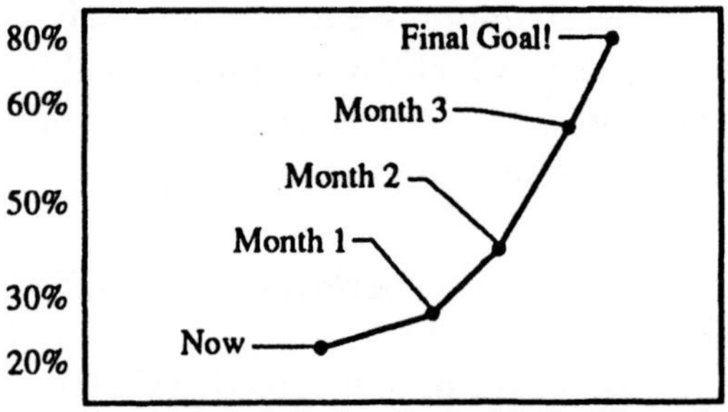

Physician Satisfaction Goals: Medical Records

uses goals will change with the situation, but the common element is that goals will become more than another poster on the wall turning yellow under fluorescent lights. They will become things to be valued and to be accomplished.

The Power of Feedback

In the daily routine of providing health care, we constantly process feedback. The nurse who administers furosemide to a critically hypertensive man anxiously monitors urine output, blood pressure, and cardiac pressures to learn whether the drug has taken effect. After administering a bronchodilator, a therapist listens to breath sounds for patient response, but also monitors vital signs to determine if there is any developing side effect. If there is positive movement toward a goal (the patient's condition improves), the clinician receives reinforcement for the value of her work. If there is no or a negative response, the clinician knows the cause of that poor performance and can take corrective or adjunct action. The same system can be developed for the work performance of a manager's staff, if the manager is prepared to apply the same rigor of monitoring and feedback that she expects of her staff.

Many managers, inundated with volumes of data and information on a daily basis, confuse the two with effective feedback. They often assume that all information is feedback. This is simply not the case. Just as the nurse who administers

Lasix does not refer to information available in an electroen-
cephalogram or deep tendon reflex for feedback, so must the
manager carefully select which information available to him can
be used to provide performance feedback. Feedback is any
information that accomplishes the following:

- It tells whether immediate performance moves one closer to
  or farther from desired goals.
- It pinpoints the cause of any directional change (with respect to achieving goals).
- It prescribes what must be done to improve performance
  and bring it closer to reaching a goal.

In general, when a manager faces inadequate performance, he draws one of several conclusions. Either the employee
needs additional training, is unmotivated, or cannot perform in
the existing work environment.

Thomas Gilbert, one of the foremost experts in the development of feedback systems, has come to a very different conclusion. He has determined that virtually every workplace problem
caused by poor performance can be improved by at least 20
percent and often up to 50 percent just by improving the quality
or frequency of performance feedback (Gilbert, 1978). Training,
one of the most expensive and frequently used performance
improvement tools, is actually one of the least frequently needed
to correct poor performance. This certainly makes the use of
systematic feedback one of the most cost-effective performance
tools in a manager's repertoire.

What makes effective feedback about performance? Feedback is effective when it:

- Pertains to a specific behavior that is the responsibility of an
  individual staff member.
- Is positive and addresses those parts of performance that are
  correct as well as those that need to improve.
- Occurs immediately upon performance by a staff member—not at the end of the shift or on Friday afternoon.

- Describes staff performance and then compares that performance to a performance goal or desired performance.
- Is multisensory, not just words or numbers. If feedback is being given on how a physical skill was performed, a physical demonstration should supplement any oral feedback. In this way, a nurse who is receiving feedback on the insertion of an intravenous line can see precisely what a supervisor means, as well as hear her words. Similarly, when providing feedback on counseling performance, the supervisor should demonstrate body language and vocal inflections used by a staff person, to re-create and pinpoint any behavior that can be improved as well as behavior executed effectively. In health care this is especially important, because the very nature of most work involves visual cues and psychomotor skill.
- Is immediately followed by positive reinforcement for an attempt at improved performance.

Many managers might question the feasibility of these guidelines, particularly in critical care and emergency situations. After all, you simply cannot risk a patient to do this. But you cannot risk *not* managing feedback in this way. Let us examine how this feedback works in even the most tense of care situations—an unexpected cardiac arrest on a general care floor. A young staff nurse, faced with her first "real code," may be assigned the task of ventilating a patient with a resuscitation bag until an airway tube is established. When a respiratory therapist or anesthesiologist arrives, the nurse is often quickly brushed aside by the anxious newcomer, who is likely part of a cardiac arrest team, with "Here, let me do that right," or words to that effect. Consequently, the nurse feels that what she did was not appropriate, but she does not know why. Was she using the wrong equipment? Was she not maintaining an airway? Was she not ventilating properly? She also feels insecure about her ability to care for patients in this situation, and if it arises again, she will likely try to find some way out of this important function. This reduces her effectiveness as a nurse and makes her much more anxious about her work.

Although a cardiac arrest is certainly an emotional situation for all involved, there are very effective ways to improve the performance of this nurse while ensuring top-notch care for the patient. When a therapist, physician, or nursing supervisor arrives to relieve the young nurse, she might say "OK, I can take over now — thanks for getting started. You were doing fine on the rate. This man is pretty heavy, isn't he? He really needs large volumes of oxygen to ventilate. Your breaths were a bit shallow. Put your hand on the bag as I squeeze it. Feel how much volume I have to move? Listen to his breath sounds as I ventilate once the way you did. Now listen to his chest as I breathe more deeply. Can you hear the difference?" This feedback can be done in most cases as a physician is preparing to intubate. It can also be given as soon as a patient is stabilized. Now the nurse understands exactly what was done properly and what needed improvement. She also has a tactile and auditory reference for proper performance. With this immediate and positive feedback, the nurse is much more likely to perform more effectively if an arrest occurs on her floor in the future.

A manager cannot be everywhere at once. It is impossible for her to assess and provide feedback on every staff member's performance. And in many cases, staff members will be using technology developed in the past six or twelve months. In these instances, a manager may not be prepared to offer feedback. Because the goal of feedback is performance improvement and not individual appraisal, the manager is not the only person who can do the job.

To ensure that a department-wide system of frequent and effective feedback is in place, the manager must see to it that all supervisors and shift leaders are also performance coaches. Performance coach is not a title bestowed upon a supervisor. It describes anyone who can provide feedback and coaching that is accepted by the staff. A manager can develop supervisors who are performance coaches by training supervisors in the process of coaching. Coaching skills include the use of feedback to improve work. They are also not magically bestowed upon individuals when they are promoted to supervisory positions. These skills must be learned and practiced. The manager must also do more than simply mandate that "all supervisors provide feedback." Supervisors must see the manager coaching and providing feedback so they understand its importance and its effectiveness. In addition, the manager can reinforce supervisors who begin using feedback on a regular basis.

Positive Reinforcement

There are three causes for poor performance in any workplace. These causes, in descending order of occurrence, are motivational problems, insufficient knowledge, and a poorly designed physical environment for work. Motivational challenges to performance are by far the most frequent and especially influential in fast-paced, highly stressful health care provider organizations. "Burnout" and "not living up to potential" are words often heard in acute care and long-term care facilities alike. In spite of the persistence of motivational problems in performance, they can be the least expensive to correct and most directly managed performance problems.

Most health care workers begin their careers highly motivated — they feel tremendous satisfaction at the prospect of being part of a humanitarian undertaking. Many also take pride in having mastered and being continuously challenged by the technologies of patient care. In short, they find their work reinforcing. The pleasure they take from their work makes them want to do it well. Unfortunately, the realities of day-to-day patient care and supporting other care givers can serve to demotivate staff. In addition to developing ways to help staff avoid and manage these demotivators, the manager must be a source of positive reinforcement for staff.

Of all the ways to improve performance, positive reinforcement is the most effective approach. Positive reinforcement is more than offering praise for jobs well done. The need for humans to receive positive reinforcement is powerful — so powerful that we constantly seek this reinforcement in all spheres of life. We choose friends and recreational activities by the amount of reinforcement we receive. We select studies and careers because of the pleasure we derive from them. Even counterproductive habits are formed essentially because of the positive reinforcement they provide. Smokers continue their habit in spite of full knowledge of its danger because they derive pleasure from smoking.

What is the difference between feedback and reinforcement? Feedback will tell someone what must be done to improve performance, and positive reinforcement will increase the likelihood that an attempt will be made to perform. So effective is positive reinforcement that many people choose to perform jobs that are poorly paying or perceived as undesirable simply because those jobs have a great deal of reinforcement associated with them. This is certainly the case of the floor nurse who continues to work the night shift in a busy hospital when she could more than double her salary by working for a pharmaceutical firm as a sales representative or for an insurance company in utilization review.

This may seem too good to be true or too simple to be effective. Managing positive reinforcement is one of the most powerful performance improvement tools available to a manager, but it is definitely not a simple tool to master. What is needed for powerful positive reinforcement? To be effective, reinforcement must be immediate, produce a performance return greater than its cost, be controlled by the manager, and be meaningful.

Reinforcement only works when it occurs immediately following performance. To offer reinforcement before a task is completed communicates to the staff that their work is done. To offer it an extended time after completion of a task may suggest that the reinforcement is for some other performance. Because feedback must be immediate to be effective, a manager must use reinforcers that are immediately available. This means that time-honored reinforcers such as annual salary increases and promotions are not as effective in reinforcing performance as those things that occur immediately after performance.

Relative value is another important aspect of positive reinforcement. Many objections to reinforcers in the workplace center on the perceived cost. Because monetary incentives and other tangible reinforcers do work, many people believe that they are expensive. The real cost of these types of incentives is in how much money is saved through increased productivity and decreased waste. An incentive system that provides bonuses costing $20,000 and only produces $10,000 in savings is very expensive. But one that costs $20,000 and produces a savings of $40,000 is a bargain. Beginning in the early 1980s and continuing to a lesser extent today, many providers experimented with tangible reinforcements to recruit professional staff. Existing staff were given such things as color televisions and cash bonuses for recruiting colleagues to work on staff. These programs often cost tens of thousands of dollars, but even greater amounts of money were saved by reducing corporate recruiting costs and increasing the capacity to generate revenue through additional staffing.

Not every manager is fortunate enough to have a budget that will allow for extensive tangible reinforcement. Nor can a manager offer a raise or promotion to every deserving staff member. To be effective for frequent use, reinforcement must come from things that a manager can control. For example, a manager who has taken the time to learn about her staff might readily be able to provide reinforcement with items of tangible value, such as a day off with pay, a journal subscription paid for from a department's petty cash fund, or a dinner and a stage show provided by the manager. Intangible reinforcement, or reinforcement with little or no monetary value, often can be more effective than the tangible variety and is more completely at the discretion of the manager. This type of reinforcement might include a simple "Thanks for a job well done" or inviting a staff member to give a report of project work to the manager's boss and other interested executives.

The notion that "one man's trash is another man's treasure" applies well to the effectiveness of reinforcement. With the exception of universally effective social reinforcers, each person will have very different responses to different methods of reinforcement. And even with such universal reinforcers as praise and paid time off, there will be a variance in how different people will perceive them. To be effective in reinforcing performance, a manager must learn what will be reinforcing to each individual staff member. How can he do this? The most effective way is to observe people in their daily routines and to listen to the casual conversation they share. The things a person chooses to do on her own are a source of effective individual reinforcers. Because a person will voluntarily do things that are reinforcing, the manager can use those things to improve performance. (For one person this might be participating in a research project. For another it might be expansion of duties to include administrative functions as well as technical. For still another it might be time off on the first day of the trout-fishing season.) How does this work in practice? One nursing manager noticed that whenever possible, one of her "floor nurses" was absorbed by the multiple electrocardiogram monitors at the nursing station. The nurse enjoyed the challenge of correctly interpreting complicated strips and spent his free time searching the monitors for unusual rhythm patterns. The manager obtained a self-paced training program in advanced electrocardiogram interpretation and made it available to the nurse contingent upon completion of basic nursing duties. The manager also spent time with the nurse, coaching his development. The result was a staff nurse who readily accepted even the most unpleasant of assignments and completed them as proficiently as possible in order to do something that was reinforcing to him.

Most managers are unfamiliar with the systematic use of positive reinforcement and so find it difficult to identify, much less use, reinforcers in such a fashion. The workplace abounds with reinforcers, though, and the trick for the manager is to match available reinforcers with appropriate individuals. Below is a list of reinforcers that are usually effective.

No- or Low-Cost Reinforcers

- Verbal praise
- Asking a staff member for an opinion or advice
- Personal notes or phone calls after extra effort such as working a double shift
- Supporting professional activities of staff: paying for conference attendance, encouraging a staff member to present

reports at symposia, providing time for committee work, donating department resources for community activities
- Providing pizza or doughnuts for volunteers who work overtime on short notice
- Job rotation
- Advanced training
- Prompt feedback on performance improvements
- Increased autonomy
- Increased individual visibility in the organization: assigning staff to interdepartmental project teams, allowing staff to present proposals and reports to administrative officers, letting staff members attend management meetings, encouraging/sponsoring a staff member's work with a medical director or other physicians for new initiatives and service development

Variable Cost Reinforcers

- Raises
- Bonuses
- Promotions
- Incentive systems that pay for innovations (for example, a fixed bonus or a percentage of revenue made/saved through cost reduction suggestions or new service developments)
- Extra paid time off
- Trips

These are only generic reinforcers used successfully in many different organizations. There are also at least as many individual-dependent reinforcers for the staff of a department. These individual-specific reinforcers are likely to be the most effective and least costly of all—but the manager must identify them.

Even the most effective reinforcer, however, will not improve performance unless it is properly managed. In fact, many managers do use reinforcers, but not so they are available contingent on performance. Indeed, this is precisely how many managers come to question the value of performance improvement. They see themselves as very supportive managers who always exude empathy and are quick with praise and a smile for their staff. They cannot understand why, when they are obviously such "nice guys," they cannot seem to get any more performance than the tyrant who runs another department. The problem with the "nice guy" manager is that indiscriminate use of reinforcers reinforces everything. Systematic performance improvement selectively reinforces only goal-oriented behavior when that behavior is measured and verified.

A more common problem than the manager who effusively reinforces at random is insufficient use of reinforcement. Many managers think they are offering adequate reinforcement for performance when in fact they are not. Behavioral research tells us that a manager should reinforce appropriate behavior at least four times for every time he punishes (reprimands, corrects, or otherwise disciplines) undesirable performance. Dr. Aubrey Daniels (1988) has collected data that ratios as high as twenty reinforcers for every punisher can be even more effective and still without risk of becoming an ineffective "nice guy" manager.

So how does one manage the delivery of effective reinforcement? There are four basic steps.

1. Use a reinforcement data system. Monitor the types of reinforcement offered to each staff member. Track each performance reinforced, the reinforcement used, and the apparent result of that reinforcement. This develops a reinforcement data base so a manager can learn precisely what reinforcers are most effective for each staff member. In addition, performances that are reinforced are available for review. This will tell the manager whether goal-directed behavior is being reinforced and with which employees. The thought of developing and maintaining such a detailed data base of management behavior may seem overwhelming to managers, but the information provided is powerful and can greatly strengthen both reinforcement effectiveness and the quality of staff performance. Exhibit 8.2 shows a sample format for a reinforcement data entry system.

2. Make sure that reinforcement is delivered immediately *after* the performance desired. To deliver reinforcement be-

Exhibit 8.2. Sample Reinforcement Log.

Date	Staff Member	Performance	Reinforcement	Response	Goal

fore the performance removes incentive for completing the performance.

3. Make sure that all managers and supervisors understand and use positive reinforcement. Prerequisite to effective reinforcement is the ability to provide it frequently and consistently for all staff members. Most staffs of health care departments are dispersed over a ward or floor. By empowering supervisors with the ability to provide staff reinforcement, a manager enriches the role of supervisor from that of overseer and problem solver to performance coach. She also increases the opportunity to provide reinforcement to all staff without having to be physically with them. A manager who does not require that all supervisors practice and use positive reinforcement on their respective shifts will certainly end up with a situation in which the majority of staff want to work only for those supervisors who do use reinforcement. This obviously creates scheduling problems.

4. Do not send mixed messages. Positive reinforcement is a powerful performance tool, but feedback, goal setting, and even punishment are also part of the world of health care management. Do not try to have a single contact with a staff member serve several of these functions. For example, a manager observing a nurse obtain blood samples from central catheters offers the following feedback: "You're doing much better at this now, but you still need some practice." This man-

ager may be trying to offer reinforcement, or he may be doing a poor job of providing specific feedback. The nurse who hears this certainly will not be terribly excited with her performance, and she will not know what to do about it. The manager will be much more effective if he deals with one issue at a time. For example, reinforcement for this situation might be to bring a new nurse to observe how one obtains a sample of blood, as demonstrated by the first nurse, or to specifically compliment those steps executed precisely. Feedback might be put in the form of questions such as "Did you flush the catheter with heparin yet?" and would be given separately from providing reinforcement.

Summary

Improving departmental performance requires that the manager assume responsibility for many of the determinants of excellence. Chapter Seven presented the most important of the manager's responsibilities for ongoing training and development. This chapter covered components of performance that can function independently of formal training and development.

Managing these components of performance involves, at a minimum, setting goals systematically, developing criterion-referenced performance expectations, and managing positive reinforcement. All of these managerial responsibilities are simple to understand but complex in their execution. The challenge for the manager is to understand the "soft and fuzzy" elements of human performance for what they really are: a controllable series of behaviors that result from titrated performance feedback and positive reinforcement. For the manager willing to exert concerted effort in performance improvement, however, there is no limit to how productive and, yes, happy her staff can be.

9
❧

From Caretaker to Leader: *Becoming a Strategic Manager*

Midlevel health care managers are being called upon to assume greater levels of responsibility and more prominent roles in the planning of services and programs for the community. This book has described why the mantle of leadership is placed on the shoulders of the health care manager, and the most important issues facing the manager-leader. By convention, the text is divided into discrete chapters, with each addressing a specific set of issues and skills for managerial effectiveness. This division, however, belies a fundamental aspect of management all too familiar to health care managers: A manager must juggle communication, projects, team building, planning, training, and hundreds of other issues simultaneously. Any of the topics presented in this book would be easier to master, if that were the exclusive focus of a manager's job, or if she had the luxury of developing the skills one set at a time, mastering each before moving on to the next. But such is not the case for most managers.

However, there are several things a manager can do to build a solid foundation for managerial excellence in each of these areas of performance. This chapter outlines six factors.

233

Expand Awareness

With so many issues facing a manager, the first question that likely comes to mind is "Where do I start?" That place is the center, and the center is you. As I have maintained throughout this book, the midlevel manager in health care is one of the most important resources available for organizational success. Given this importance of the manager, he must be viewed as a precious commodity in which investments must be made for continual renewal. As that manager, the most immediate investment you can make is to consciously and constantly increase your awareness of the facets of the health care industry that are the furthest from your own professional expertise. Consciously reviewing industry periodicals in management, finance, marketing, and technical arenas, as well as business periodicals, provides the information a manager needs to build a vision of what is possible and to communicate and defend that vision to others.

Build a Foundation of Trust

Strengthening your awareness of the industry of health care is a process that you can start immediately, but never really complete. Fulfilling the leader's obligation to maintaining trust is also like this. Of the six functions of a leader, the most important to the success of the others is maintaining trust. Without this, a leader's followers will not share her vision, trust her judgment, or follow willingly. Trust is also one of the few responsibilities of the health care manager that is exclusively the result of the manager's behavior. The continual process of becoming a health care leader must begin by establishing and maintaining a positive trust between the manager and every person and department with whom she interacts.

Few would argue that awareness and trust are not essential for effective health care leaders. Perhaps the most significant departure today's manager must make with tradition, though, is in how he perceives himself within the organization. A few years ago, successful managers in health care, if asked, would have said that the secret to success is conscientious management of operations.

Become a Spark

Today, though, the greatest contribution a manager can make to an organization is to empower those around him to excel. Managers who do this effectively do not see themselves as managers of operations, but they recognize the role they play as sparks, igniting fires of creativity and accomplishment in the people around them. Managing operations becomes secondary in personal importance for the health care leader. This funda- mental shift in self-perception is a difficult one for many health care managers to make—and yet it is essential to the ability of a leader to lead.

Operations continue to receive close attention, but the manager who is a spark finds creative ways to manage those operations. He constantly looks for opportunities to share this part of his job with supervisors and staff. Delegation, project assignments, and other strategies are used to spread the respon- sibilities around. How do staff react to this? When done effec- tively, they see these responsibilities as expanding the scope of their influence over the department and as a sign of trust that the manager would share the power of his position. What the manager also accomplishes is creating more time to focus on being a spark and on becoming a leader.

Build a Framework for Effective Communication

This framework begins by establishing an environment of positive trust within the department. This facet of effective communication is so essential that it bears repeating. It will also take time and patience if this trust does not already exist. When trust is established, a structural framework can be built and added to as time passes. This framework should include at least two elements that a manager can put in place without undue organizational effort:

- Establish a formal structure that provides opportunities for both group and one-on-one communication among the manager, supervisors, and department staff. Commit to this structure and do not deviate from it.
- Lead by example. The manager's influence upon his department is only as good as the example he sets. To create an environment of effective communication for problem solving and teamwork, a manager must initiate the process by actively seeking and demonstrably heeding input from supervisors and staff. This is not without challenge or risk, as the manager who invites input and constructive criticism is admitting that he does not always have all of the answers. Although this is a simple fact of life, it can be very threatening on a personal level to managers who are not secure in their leadership ability.

With these structures in place, managers can then focus on communication as the *vehicle* it is for idea exchange, problem solving, and mutual support, rather than as the *substance* of an issue to be managed.

Adopt a Planning Attitude

The essence of this book's message about planning is much simpler than the specific strategies and procedures described in Chapter Four. Successful managers realize that the most important aspect of planning is its relevance to the organization. You must be able to relate the value of planned efforts directly to the provider organization. This is certainly in part the result of logical analysis and effective communication. But more to the point is the manager's attitude that the time and energy of his department are far too important to spend in activities that do not in some way improve the overall organization.

Before successful managers ever worry about the detailed process of planning, they ask themselves several questions:

- What are the most important things that this organization is trying to accomplish?

- What is the greatest contribution we can make to those things?
- What will it look like when we are successful? (How will things be different?)

These questions are similar to the description of the manager's responsibility as a leader to be a visionary. The most important part of planning for health care managers is the vision of success driving that planning. This is the kernel of planning that should be the starting point for effective managers. Many leaders have observed that this vision, if clear enough and shared by all involved, can provide guidance to compensate for other weaknesses in the planning process. If this vision is developed, the manager can then apply specific planning strategies and employ precise tools as they become relevant to realizing that vision, rather than trying to master all of the skills of systematic planning at once.

Focus on the Performance System

Much of this book addressed the "people" side of effective management, from team building and project management to improving staff performance through training and other performance systems. The reason for this emphasis is uncomplicated. The only way a manager succeeds is through "her people" — the staff and others who contribute time and energy actually doing the work that she manages. The tools provided in these chapters are powerful and will work. But they are only tools. To use these tools most effectively, the manager must view the provider organization as a total system whose function is performance.

Most health care managers are well acquainted with a systems model. Allied health managers in particular have studied living systems for many years. They accept that it is essential for a clinician to understand the function of one system and its interactions with other systems in order to treat a patient. For example, to treat acidemia, one must understand how the pulmonary, renal, and circulatory systems interact with each other to create and alleviate the condition. This understanding allows

the clinician to prescribe precise interventions to create a desired effect on the system. The performance of a provider organization is analogous in many ways to the physical system of the
human body. By understanding the different subsystems *within*
that system, and the interactions of each, the manager can
strengthen performance within the system as specifically and
reliably as clinicians strengthen the performance of the body.
Just as the health of a person can be objectively assessed, and
specific interventions prescribed to improve that health, so too
can a manager diagnose and prescribe interventions for performance improvement.

To become a performance manager, though, the health
care manager must first step back from the operation of the
system that is his department and understand the components
of performance that make it work. These components, like the
components of the body, all serve primary functions. When the
manager understands the function of each component, he will
understand the role they play in organizational success. Only
then should he concern himself with the appropriate use of the
detailed strategies and tools described in this text.

How does a manager approach the performance system?
The case in Resource D demonstrates one manager's approach
to meeting the needs of the performance system. In this example
the manager moves through a process of planning, communicating, problem solving, and performance improvement that
uses nearly all of the strategies described in this text. His approach is driven by the strategic needs of the organization and
the performance needs of the people of the organization. This
example focuses on a manager in a human resources capacity,
but the systematic application of these tools is effective in all
areas of the provider. Exhibit II in the case is a component of the
Quan-Com™ Selection System, which was researched, developed, and validated by Donald N. Lombardi and CHR/Inter-
vista, Inc. The Quan-Com model and this tool are described in
detail in the *Handbook of Personnel Selection and Performance Evaluation in Healthcare* (Lombardi, 1988).

Throughout this book I have focused on presenting issues
that are essential for managers in health care to bridge the gap

between administrative management and true leadership in an industry that can no longer wait for dynamic leaders. Many of the issues addressed are often discussed in management meetings and retreats. And on occasion department managers are invited by executives to attend these meetings. The difference between a leader and a nonleader is in how these issues are addressed and how the skills of leadership are practiced and honed. Leaders in the health care industry will apply the concepts and procedures that are captured in this book, bringing them to life in daily practice. Others, who choose not to lead, will simply read and consider the issues as interesting concepts for discussion or debate.

Be a leader. Address the issues presented here within whatever scope your position allows. Practice the skills presented, whether you manage a single service or department or have several managers working for you.

Resource A
Competency Areas for Health Care Managers

Senior Management

I. Technical Skills
  A. *Skill Cluster: Corporate Management*
    This cluster includes those areas used to manage business risks in maximizing organizational performance. Component Skill Areas:
    • Management of a Portfolio of Businesses
    • Business Risk Evaluation (Risk Taking)
    • Management of Alternative Business Structures (HMOs, limited partnerships)
    • Evaluation of Product Life Cycles
    • Establish Incentives for Individual and Organizational Performance
    • Management of Business Development Within Available Resources
    • Management of Corporate Marketing and Sales Processes

Source: Stevens, 1987b.

240

    B.   *Skill Cluster: Financial Management Skills*
       This cluster includes all accounting, financial management, and investment management skills.
       Component Skill Areas:
- General Financial Management Skills
- Investment Management Skills
- Ability to Explain, Analyze, and Manage Insurance Functions

II.   Communicative Skills

    A.   *Skill Cluster: Managing Uncertainty*
       This cluster contains those skill areas critical to managing organizational change, as well as definition and management of previously unknown system variables.
       Component Skill Areas:
- Skill at Directing Change Management
- Managing Interdependence/Delegation
- Ability to Use Analytical and Intuitive Decision-Making Processes
- Ability to Define and Solve Problems

    B.   *Skill Cluster: Use of Influence*
       This cluster contains all skill areas whose purpose is to communicate to and direct the behavior of people or organizations.
       Component Skill Areas:
- Human Relations Management
- Media and Presentation Forum Communications
- Political Influence
- Listening Skills
- Communication of Corporate Values to Staff and Business Partners
- Skill at Negotiation

III.   Organizational/Industry Knowledge

    A.   *Intimate Understanding of Critical Industry Issues*
- Development of New Corporate Organizational Structures to Oversee Divergent Activities of Providers
- Development of Corporate Organizational Strat-

egies to Implement Divergent Activities of Providers
- Effective Human Resource Management
- Development of Alternatives in Acquiring Business Capital
- Development of Ongoing Systems of Assessment of the Business Environment and Analysis of Its Impact upon Organizational Plans
- Physician Relationships with Provider Organizations

Midlevel Management Executives

I. Technical Skills
- Departmental Cost Control
- Productivity Management
- Operations Management Under Prospective Payment
- Marketing Health Care Services
- Development/Implementation of Performance Standards
II. Communicative Skills
- Defining and Using Group Problem-Solving Processes
- Interpersonal Communication
- Conflict Resolution
- Change Management
III. Organizational/Industry Knowledge
- Prospective Payment Systems
- Innovative Services Offered in Health Care

Resource B

A Competency Worksheet

Competency	Weight			x	Score			= Total
	Critical/New	Important	Nice to Have	x	Needs Improvement	Adequate	Outstanding Masters	=
	1	2	3		1	2	3	

Resource C

An Individual Development Plan

PERSONAL HISTORY

Employee Name (last, first & initial)	Date of Birth	Emp No.	Date Employed

Colleges/Universities	Major(s)	Degree(s)	Year(s)

(list earliest experience first)

Division	Position	Reporting to	Date Assigned

Out-of-Company Educational/Training Programs	Year

Intra-Company Training Programs	Year

Previous Work or Other Experience Related to Position

Organization	Position/Rank	Dates From	To

Current Information

Division	Department	Position	Position Level	Management Skill Rating	PMS Eval. Date

Current Assignment (Describe major elements, including unique responsibilities)

Strengths (personal attributes and abilities: give examples)			

Opportunities to use strengths on the job			

Employee Development Needs

Developmental Needs	Development Plan to Meet Needs	Plans for using skills on the job	Timetable

Recent development experiences accomplished (indicate date completed)

Employee's Preferences **for future assignments**

Employee's Preferences .	Management's Recommendations to Employee

Possible **future assignments (functions/projects/positions)**

	Date

Additional Comments

SIGNATURES

Employee	Date
Manager	Date

Sample Skill Inventory

Review the following list of skills and rank each skill using a scale as follows:

4	3	2	1
Very High	Above Average	Average	Low

Rate: (A) The level of skill needed to be effective in your current position.
(B) The level of skill you demonstrate in your current position.

Skills may be rated by several individuals to provide you with additional input and feedback (for example, manager, peer, and subordinate).

	Level of skill needed in current position:								Level of skill demonstrated in current position:							
	Self Rating				Mgr. Rating				Self Rating				Mgr. Rating			
	4	3	2	1	4	3	2	1	4	3	2	1	4	3	2	1
PLANNING WORK																
• Sets and meets measurable short-term goals using a systematic and collaborative approach.																
• Sets and meets measurable long-range goals using a systematic and collaborative approach.																
• Adequately researches resources, data, and activity of concurrent projects prior to developing plans.																
• Effectively consults with appropriate levels of management to assess available resources/information necessary to deliver quality project/product.																
• Has a thorough knowledge of business operations and procedures to adequately assess the impact of their unit/project on corporate goals and objectives.																
• Analyzes and presents in advance the costs/benefits of programs/projects.																
• Analyzes current and future trends, anticipates changes, and develops alternatives and contingency plans.																
• Develops priorities and sequences issues and tasks to meet corporate goals.																
• Plans for improved productivity and quality performance.																
• Researches and collects data and formulates plans and recommendations.																

	Level of skill needed in current position:				Level of skill demonstrated in current position:			
	Self Rating		Mgr. Rating		Self Rating		Mgr. Rating	
	4 3 2 1		4 3 2 1		4 3 2 1		4 3 2 1	
• Develops budgets, forecasts, and systems for operational planning purposes (year to year) that support the corporation's long-range plans.								
•								
•								
•								
CONTROLLING WORK								
• Manages and controls administrative functions to include documentation, budget maintenance, and performance appraisal.								
• Monitors quality and quantity of work consistently and in a timely manner.								
• Monitors and updates the cost/benefits information of programs/projects.								
• Evaluates results, modifies plans, and assesses contingencies to meet goals/ results.								
•								
•								
•								
CLIMATE SETTING								
• Establishes clear and measurable standards of performance.								
• Maintains high productivity while fostering high employee morale.								
• Creates an open climate that fosters cooperative effort, collaboration, and teamwork.								
• Provides and encourages new, creative solutions to problems.								
• Responds to pressure and manages stress in a way that minimizes negative effect in the work environment.								
• Uses power and authority in a positive way.								
• Improves work procedures, methods, and systems.								
• Exhibits flexibility and adaptability to change.								

	Level of skill needed in current position:								Level of skill demonstrated in current position:							
	Self Rating				Mgr. Rating				Self Rating				Mgr. Rating			
	4	3	2	1	4	3	2	1	4	3	2	1	4	3	2	1
• Advances the image of the corporation internally/externally through speeches, consultations, and other oral/written communications with employees, subscribers, providers, and the general public.																
•																
•																
•																
DELEGATING																
• Appropriately selects tasks to be delegated.																
• Achieves results by effectively working through subordinates and others.																
• Gives clear and precise directions when assigning work.																
• Assesses strengths, values, goals, and development needs of staff and demonstrates knowledge of resources available to address each.																
• Encourages and uses subordinate solutions to problems.																
• Encourages and uses high level of involvement in the decision-making process.																
•																
•																
•																

After completing your analysis in all categories (Planning, Controlling, Climate Set-ting, and Delegating), review your ratings to make sure they reflect your best judg-ments. Then total each general category and fill in the appropriate distribution boxes for both Column A and Column B below. Use both the individual ratings and the general totals for comparison between self and manager and/or others.

General Category	Self-Rating Totals		Manager Rating Totals	
	Needed	Demonstrated	Needed	Demonstrated
Planning				
Controlling				
Climate Setting				
Delegating				

Resource D
Case Study: Parkston Memorial Hospital

The following case demonstrates how a manager at Parkston Memorial Hospital successfully handled the development of competencies in management staff using a top-down, or general to specific, model of training and development planning.

Scenario

Parkston Hospital Authority (PHA) is a small not-for-profit, multi-institutional system providing health care services to a metropolitan area of 255,000 and fifteen suburban and rural communities of 750 to 2,600 people in a 200-mile geographic diameter. The hub of this system are two hospitals of 400 and 200 beds with four satellite centers providing surgical, obstetrical, family practice, elder-care, and home care services to its communities. Parkston's current competition includes a 300-bed not-for-profit hospital with competing satellite service networks and a recently opened for-profit hospital of 220 beds with specialized satellite centers for ambulatory surgical care (see Figure D.1).

Three years ago, Parkston's board hired a new CEO and COO in hopes of turning around the system's faltering financial performance (losses at that time were $1.8 million for the fiscal year). In the ensuing three years, Parkston's performance has significantly improved. With a net annual balance of $2.4 million, the CEO and COO feel that they have turned the corner. Many of the key managers at Parkston who have been instrumental in this turnaround have been promoted (often to replace their former managers who have "sought other career opportunities") and have learned quickly the need to work together as a management team. Seven of these sixteen managers are new to the field of hospital administration; they were formerly department heads in nursing, radiology, and surgery, as well as mid-level administrative support personnel.

Project Rationale

Recognizing that sustained long-term growth will require consistent, dynamic leadership from the young administrative staff, the COO has recommended to his CEO that a program of intensive training be instituted. The CEO, Sarah Thompson, has completely endorsed the concept and has dubbed the plan "Project Space Camp," which she feels embodies the forward-thinking, elite group of leaders who should be the result of this project. Thompson also recognizes the importance of bringing the young managers of the corporation together with more senior staff and industry experts to:

- Provide younger managers with the perspective of senior managers regarding Parkston's history. She hopes this will help her team avoid repetition of past errors.
- Provide senior managers with concentrated exposure to the energy and ideas of younger managers.
- Develop a unified vision of Parkston's direction for the future.
- Develop the skills necessary in a management staff to successfully compete in a corporatized industry.

Figure D.1. Map of Parkston Hospital Authority Service Area.

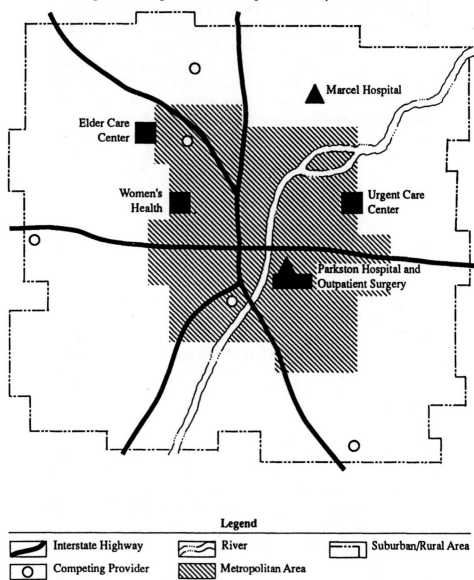

Exhibit D.1. Summary of Interview Conducted with COO
Strategic Plan Goals and Component Objectives.

Goal I: Achieve corporate growth through implementation of new services.

Objectives:

I.1   PHA will provide 70 percent of all elder-care services delivered in its market area within five years.

I.2   PHA will continue to provide 15 percent of its inpatient care to those unable to pay for these services.

I.3   Fifty percent of PHA's revenue will be from sources outside of inpatient care.

Goal II: Reduce operating expenses associated with inefficiency by 50 percent (those costs not associated with either billable services or facility maintenance). This means reductions in managerial staff levels.

Objectives:

II.1   Increase managerial efficiency through position modification to provide increased financial and market development responsibility to administrative staff.

II.2   Eliminate marginally productive management positions and reassign or outplace position incumbents.

II.3   Identify and implement specific methods for improving resource allocation and utilization efficiency in materials (expendables), capital equipment, and nonpatient-care personnel.

Definition of Strategic Priorities

John Valiant, director of human resources, is consulted on the development of the program. Being a practical man, he recognizes that organizational business plans and the culture engendered in the leadership styles of executive management need to serve as the foundation for constructing an effective leadership development program. Exhibit D.1 summarizes Valiant's interview with the COO. The leadership styles of the CEO and COO, while subjectively apparent to Valiant, were quantitatively verified using the management style profile system in use at Parkston. The results of this profile also follow as Exhibit D.2.

The Quan-Com Selection System traits listed below are determined through an open interview in which the candidate demonstrates via his experiences reliance upon critical management and leadership skills. The degree of trait use is quantified by trained interviewers and compared to organizational/job requirements. (See Lombardi, 1988, for more information about Quan-Com.)

I. *Attitude Orientation*
1. *Adaptability*—Proven ability to perform well under changing conditions, high stress, and adverse physical conditions; can relate to varied personalities, and absorb new methods with excellent practical results.
2. *Aggressiveness*—Takes command appropriately in all situations; enterprising, direct, and effectively persuasive in all business dealings.
3. *Perseverance*—Pursues established work schedule and goals tirelessly to a successful end despite any situational obstacles; willing to go the distance every time.
4. *Work Ethic*—Displays a consistently sound attitude and a positive "can do" approach to all situations; manifests a realistic aura of being capable and ready to perform any tasks that will contribute to the good of the organization.

II. *People Skills*
1. *Communication*—Can express needs and desires effectively to co-workers and superiors in a professional manner; deals tactfully but advantageously with external parties.
2. *Energy Level*—Displays a steady, fast pace in executing assignments, and an innate ability to increase activity to the maximum when necessary; possesses suitable vitality and endurance for present and future assignments.
3. *Perceptiveness*—Has a comprehensive understanding of the human quotient as it relates to the workplace; good dexterity in both internal and external interpersonal dealings.
4. *Presence/Bearing*—Creates a positive impression and makes his presence known in any given situation with favorable results.

Exhibit D.2. The Selection Proformance:™ Quan-Com™ Scoresheet.

Candidate _____ Phone _____

Address _____

Company _____ Interviewer _____

Position _____ Interview Date _____

Orig. copy   —
Canary copy   —
0 = Marginal • 1 = Satisfactory • 2 = Strong Evidence   Pink copy   — Chr.

1. Performs well under changing circum-stances, high stress, or adverse physical conditions; can absorb different processes and new methods with practicality.	INTERVIEWER NOTES:	Adaptability	
2. Commits to hard work for the organization, consistently representing its best interest by giving its needs top priority; intrinsic dedication to cause and duty.		Loyalty	
3. Pursues work tirelessly to a successful completion despite obstacles; willing to go the distance consistently.		Perseverance	
4. Displays a sound, positive attitude and a "can do" approach; capable and ready to perform for the good of the organization.		Work Ethic	
	ATTITUDE ORIENTATION	Subtotal	
1. Can express needs and desires to co-workers and superiors appropriately; deals courteously and tactfully with external parties.	INTERVIEWER NOTES:	Communication	
2. Displays a steady, fast pace consistently and an ability to increase activity effectively as necessary. Suitable vitality and endurance.		Energy Level	
3. Willing to discuss situations and circumstances, consistently honest, candid, and direct. Does not harbor needed information.		Openness	
	INTERPERSONAL TRAITS	Subtotal	
1. Ability to analyze quantitative and qualitative data and make logical determinations and educated perceptions; pragmatically applies intellect to the work situation.	INTERVIEWER NOTES:	Raw Intelligence	
2. Possesses an adequate range of appropriate experience with similar responsibilities thereby providing a realistic frame of reference.		Work Experience	
	PROFORMANCE QUALIFICATIONS	Subtotal	

1. Highly motivated toward selfless service toward co-workers, customers, and organizational goals; looks at tasks as a commitment to others and organizational excellence.	INTERVIEWER NOTES:	Cooperation	
2. Capable of ascertaining direction and goals, self-starting; can make judgments, decisions, and executions without much reliance on others.		Indep. Motivation	
3. Demonstrates poise and self-confidence to assume tasks and responsibilities appropriately; accepts responsibility and produces on a timely basis.		Responsiveness	
	TEAM ORIENTATION	Subtotal	
© 1984		TOTAL SCORE	

Optional additional demographic data to be completed after decision based on employee records and applicant flow data for validation purposes only.

(1) _____ (4) _____   REJECTED ☐
(2) _____ (5) _____   ACCEPTED ☐
(3) _____ Position __   HIRED ☐

With an understanding of where Parkston was going in the next five years, Valiant began the next step in developing the leadership program for the system: the definition of key issues for program content with subsequent definition of priority target audiences by position title. The PHA organizational chart shown in Exhibit D.3 demonstrates the organizational levels encompassed in this initial effort.

Definition of Leadership Issues

To define the most important issues facing management, Valiant opted to conduct a nominal group session at a management meeting for PHA because a consensus of priorities affecting all PHA subsidiaries was needed. The management meeting was attended by all corporate staff and the administrators of all subsidiaries.

Exhibit D.3. Parkston Hospital Authority Management Structure.

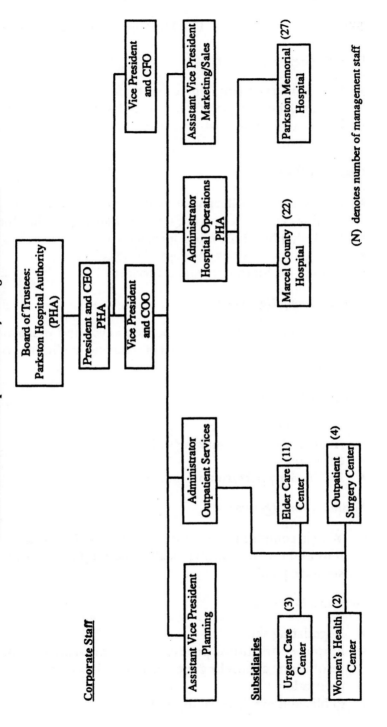

Corporate Staff

Board of Trustees: Parkston Hospital Authority (PHA)

President and CEO PHA

Vice President and CFO

Assistant Vice President Marketing/Sales

Vice President and COO

Administrator Hospital Operations PHA

Parkston Memorial Hospital (27)

Marcel County Hospital (22)

Assistant Vice President Planning

Administrator Outpatient Services

Elder Care Center (11)

Outpatient Surgery Center (4)

Subsidiaries

Urgent Care Center (3)

Women's Health Center (2)

(N) denotes number of management staff

Nominal Group Question 1:

- Which management skills, other than communication/feed-back, will be most helpful to you and your staff in achieving the strategic plan goals of growth through development of new services?

Consensus Priorities:

- Management of alternative delivery systems — for example, satellite centers, home care services, housing for the elderly
- Marketing health care products/services
- Competitive business strategy
- Sales of health care products/services

Nominal Group Question 2:

- Which skills will be most important to you and your staff in achieving PHA's strategic goal of reducing inefficiency costs by 50 percent?

Consensus Priorities:

- Financial management
- Analytical/decision-making skills
- Creativity
- Productivity/performance management

Nominal Group Question 3:

- Which communicative/interpersonal skills will be most important to management staff in accomplishing the PHA strategic plan?

Consensus Priorities:

- Negotiating skills
- Employee relations: productivity improvement, conflict resolution, counseling performance improvement, and motivation
- Public and media speaking skills

Nominal Group Question 4:

- What will be the greatest change in the health care delivery environment that affects PHA in the next five years?

Consensus Priorities:

- Patient population in hospitals is not increasing, and competition for outpatient care is increasing.
- Payer reimbursement (insurance payments) to hospitals for health care will not increase.
- Health care is being redefined from "curing disease" to "providing services for specific market segments," such as the "women's segment" and the "elderly segment."

Definition of Program Audience

Given this considerable list of issues facing the management of PHA, Valiant next decided to provide this feedback from the management staff to the COO of the system. This was done with two objectives in mind: (1) to receive executive input and approval regarding the potential impact of the strategic plan upon the leadership programs being planned and (2) to define the positions within PHA that would compose the program audience. Because the list of issues was long, Valiant also chose to recommend that "Project Space Camp" be a series of events rather than a single conference. To explain this recommendation clearly, Valiant presented to the COO a summary of the nominal group's findings and the following chart of development experiences for the people involved:

	Technical Skills	Communicative Skills	Industry Skills
Experience 1	Priority 1	Priority 1	Priority 1
Experience 2	Priority 2	Priority 2	Priority 2
Experience 3	Priority 3	Priority 3	Priority 3

In asking the COO to select those positions within PHA that would be priorities for a target audience, Valiant requested that the COO also consider other managers in the organization whose management style would complement those of the CEO and COO (see Exhibit D.4).

The COO authorized the development of a pilot program for the curriculum of leadership development, with authorization for further development contingent upon the pilot's success. The target audience that Valiant selected for the program, after the COO's input, follows.

The specific content areas for the project, derived from PHA strategic priorities, are shown in three categories in Exhibit D.5. These categories are technical skills of importance to the target audience, priority communicative skills, and strategically relevant industry knowledge components.

Indicators of Program Success

After defining the program, and sharing this with the executive office, Valiant set about defining acceptable standards for measuring the degree of program success. Because it was consistent with PHA's structure of management by objectives, Valiant, in discussion with the executive office, proposed that appropriate measures of skill transfer by participants be used to evaluate the program and used as objectives for program participants in their performance appraisals.

These criteria for success were selected:

- Program participants would develop functional first drafts of market development plans for each operational area represented by a corporate officer. Where market development plans currently existed, revised drafts reflecting new strategic plans would be prepared.
- Given corporate assistance, program participants would revise market plan drafts and implement both market development plans and the support communication plans produced in the conference within six months. (This criterion would be used to evaluate the program and its participants in their performance appraisals.)

Exhibit D.4. Parkston Hospital Authority Leadership Development Target Audience.

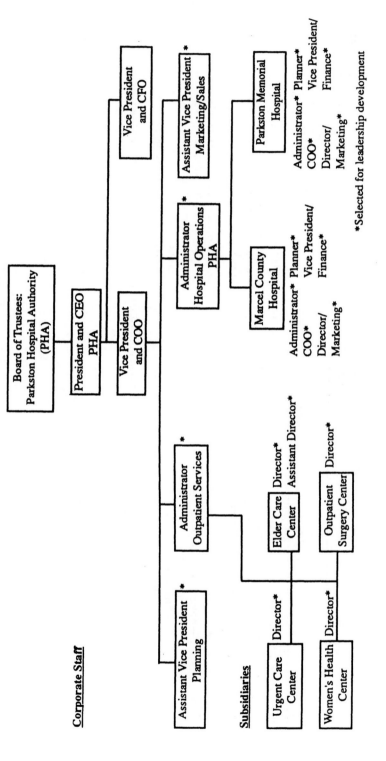

**Exhibit D.5. Program Content Areas
PHA Leadership Development.**

	Technical Area	Communicative Area	Organizational/Industry Knowledge Area
Experience 1	Market Development — the marketing process — market plan development — market plan implementation	Management Communications — formal presentation — feedback	Market Trends — national (present-future) — service area (present-future) — PHA

Experience 2	Competitive Strategy
	— competitor analysis
	— risk analysis
	  — financial
	  — business
		Negotiating Skills	Analysis of Change in the Health Care Industry
			— comparison to other industries: (banking)
			— comparison of the PHA area's change to the nation
			— analysis of PHA's response to change

Experience 3	Financial Control — finance for nonfinancial executives — cost control strategy	Public/Media Communications	Emerging Technologies in Health Care

- Anonymous participant feedback would indicate skill enhancement in communicative areas addressed.
- Training development would conduct an opinion survey of institutional staff to assess follow-up changes in managerial communication effectiveness.

References

Appelbaum, S. H. *Stress Management for Healthcare Professionals.* Rockville, Md.: Aspen Systems, 1981.

Arthur Andersen & Co. and American College of Healthcare Executives. *The Future of Healthcare: Changes and Choices.* Chicago: American College of Healthcare Executives, 1987.

Barr, L., and Barr, N. *The Leadership Equation.* Austin, Tex.: Eaken Press, 1989.

Blake, R., and Mouton, J. S. *The New Managerial Grid.* Houston, Tex.: Gulf Publishing Co., 1988.

Block, P. *Flawless Consulting: A Guide to Getting Your Expertise Used.* San Diego, Calif.: University Associates, 1981.

Block, R. *The Politics of Projects.* New York: Yourdon Press, 1983.

Bogden, R., and Taylor, S. *Introduction to Qualitative Methods.* New York: Wiley, 1975.

Bowsher, J. *Educating America: Lessons Learned in the Nation's Corporations.* New York: Wiley, 1989.

Brown-Carlson Listening Comprehension Test. Yonkers-on-Hudson, World Book Company.

Burke, D. R. *What Managers Do.* Philadelphia, Penn.: American Management Association, 1978.

Cook, T., and Reichardt, C. (eds.). *Qualitative and Quantitative Methods in Evaluation.* Newbury Park, Calif.: Sage, 1979.

Daniels, A., and Rosen, T. *Performance Management: Improving Quality and Productivity Through Positive Reinforcement.* Tucker, Ga.: Performance Management Publications, 1984.

Darr, K., Longest, B., and Rakich, J. "The Ethical Imperative in Health Services Governance and Management." *Hospital & Health Services Administration,* Mar./Apr. 1986, pp. 53–66.

de Jaager, G. *The Project Manager's Tool Kit: The Practical Guide to Successful Project Execution.* Palo Alto, Calif.: Seiler-Doar Books, 1988.

Drucker, P. *The Effective Executive.* New York: Harper & Row, 1985a.

Drucker, P. *Innovation and Enterprise.* New York: Harper & Row, 1985b.

Drucker, P. *New Realities.* New York: Harper & Row, 1989.

Ganong, J., and Ganong, W. *Nursing Management.* Rockville, Md.: Aspen Systems, 1980.

Garfield, C. *Peak Performers: The New Heroes of American Business.* New York: Avon, 1987.

Geneen, H. *Managing.* New York: Doubleday, 1984.

Goldsmith, S. *Theory Z Hospital Management: Lessons from Japan.* Rockville, Md.: Aspen Systems, 1984.

Haimann, T. *Supervisory Management for Healthcare Institutions.* St. Louis, Mo.: Catholic Hospital Press, 1973.

Hartley, R. *Management Mistakes.* Columbus, Ohio: Grid, 1983.

Hastings, C., and others. *The Superteam Solution: Successful Team-working in Organisations.* Hants, England: Gower Publishing Co., 1986.

Hunsaker, P., and Allesandra, A. *The Art of Managing People.* New York: Simon & Schuster, 1980.

Hutchison, C. "The Care and Feeding of a Network." *Performance & Instruction,* 1988, *27* (8), 17–20.

Jung, C. G. *Psychological Types.* Princeton, N.J.: Princeton University Press, 1976.

Kaufman, K., and Hall, M. "Capital Planning in Not-for-Profit Healthcare." Unpublished papers, Kaufman-Hall Associates, Northfield, Ill., 1987.

Kraut, R. (ed.). *Technology and the Transformation of White-Collar Work.* Hillsdale, N.J.: Erlbaum, 1987.

Lee, I. "Procedure for 'Coercing' Agreement." *Harvard Business Review*, 1957.

Likert, R., and Likert, J. G. *New Ways of Managing Conflict*. New York: McGraw-Hill, 1976.

Linneman, R., and Charan, R. "Contingency Planning: A Key to Swift Managerial Action in the Uncertain Tomorrow." *Managerial Planning*, Jan./Feb. 1981, pp. 23–27.

Lombardi, D. N. Unpublished market survey conducted by CHR/Intervista, Hackettstown, N.J., 1984.

Lombardi, D. N. *The Quan-Com Selection Series*. Costa Mesa, Calif.: Center for Human Resources Press, 1985.

Lombardi, D. N. *Handbook of Personnel Selection and Performance Evaluation in Healthcare*. San Francisco: Jossey-Bass, 1988.

MacGregor, D. *The Professional Manager*. New York: McGraw-Hill, 1967.

Mackenzie, A. *How to Set Priorities*. Listen, USA, 1988.

Martin, W. B. *Quality Customer Service*. Los Altos, Calif.: Crisp Publications, 1987.

Martinez, C. "How to Make Instructional Presentations." *Performance & Instruction*, 1988, *27* (3), 6–8.

Miller, L. *American Spirit: Visions of a New Corporate Culture*. New York: Warner, 1984.

Mohr, W., and Mohr, H. *Quality Circles: Changing Images of People at Work*. Reading, Mass.: Addison-Wesley, 1983.

Moskal, W. *Team Achievement Process*. Chicago: American College of Healthcare Executives Courseware, 1986.

Myers-Briggs, I., and McCauley, M. *Manual: A Guide to the Development and Use of the Myers-Briggs Type Indicator*. Palo Alto, Calif.: Consulting Psychologists Press, 1985.

Naisbitt, J., and Aburdene, P. *Re-inventing the Corporation: Transforming Your Job and Your Company for the New Information Society*. New York: Warner, 1985.

Nichols, R., and Stevens, L. "The Busy Executive Spends 80% of His Time . . . Listening to People . . . and Still Doesn't Hear Half of What Is Said." *Harvard Business Review*, 1957, pp. 85–92.

Page-Jones, M. *Practical Project Management*. New York: Dorset House, 1985.

Peters, T., and Waterman, R. *In Search of Excellence: Lessons from America's Best-Run Companies*. New York: Harper & Row, 1984.

Professional Training Associates. *Practical Supervision*. Round Rock, Tex.: Professional Training Associates, 1987.

Randolph, W., and Posner, B. *Effective Project Planning and Management: Getting the Job Done*. Englewood Cliffs, N.J.: Prentice-Hall, 1988.

Seiwert, L. J. *Time Is Money, Save It!* Homewood, Ill.: Dow-Jones Irwin, 1989.

Shelby, S. "A Macro Theory of Management Communication." *Journal of Business Communication*, Spring 1988.

Sisty, J. "International Plant Engineering Conference." In W. Weiss (ed.), *Supervisor's Standard Reference Handbook*. Englewood Cliffs, N.J.: Prentice-Hall, 1987.

Steinmatz, L. *The Art and Skill of Delegation*. Reading, Mass.: Addison-Wesley, 1976.

Stevens, G. H. "The Leadership Imperative: Defining and Building Visionary Leaders in the Healthcare Industry." Paper presented at the 25th annual conference of the National Society for Performance and Instruction, San Antonio, Tex., 1987a.

Stevens, G. H. "Needs Assessment for the American College of Healthcare Executives Affiliates, Members, and Fellows." Unpublished management strategy document, American College of Healthcare Executives, Chicago, 1987b.

Stogdill, R. M. *Handbook of Leadership*. New York: Free Press, 1974.

Svenson, R., and Wallace, K. "Performance Technology: A Strategic Management Tool." *Performance & Instruction*, 1989, *28* (8).

Takezawa, S., and Whitehall, A. *Work Ways: Japan and America*. Tokyo: Japan Institute of Labor, 1981.

Taylor, H. *Delegate: The Key to Successful Management*. New York: Beaufort, 1984.

Zuboff, S. *In the Age of the Smart Machine: The Future of Work and Power*. New York: Basic Books, 1988.

Index

Lightning Source UK Ltd.
Milton Keynes UK
29 March 2011

169992UK00002BA/1/P